"GERMS" OF TRUTH

- If antibiotics can't kill the cold and flu virus, why are they often prescribed? (See page 28.)
- How long can mayonnaise linger in the refrigerator? (See page 122.)
- Which room in your home harbors the most germs? (See page 108.)
- When should children get vaccinated for rubella? (See page 210.)
- Most colds arrive in winter. Right? (See page 76.)
- How hot should your food be served? (See page 137.)

"A practical guide to mankind's microscopic nemesis—the germ. Crammed full of authoritative answers to common questions, this book is a must-read for understanding everything from the difference between good and bad germs to the true meaning of 'organic' to the unseen terrors of biological warfare."

—Charlotte Bell, M.D., associate professor,
Yale University School of Medicine

"To read this book is to obtain a license to thrive in a world strikingly dominated by bacteria, viruses, and other unseen beasties."

—Moselio Schaechter, Ph.D., professor emeritus,
Tufts University School of Medicine

D0816260

Don't Touch That Doorknob!

How germs can zap you and how you can zap back

jack brown,
ph.d.

WARNER BOOKS

A Time Warner Company

Copyright © 2001 by John C. Brown, Ph.D. and Byron Preiss Visual Publications, Inc.
All rights reserved.

Warner Books, Inc., 1271 Avenue of the Americas, New York, NY 10020
Visit our Web site at www.twbookmark.com.
For information on Time Warner Trade Publishing's online publishing program, visit www.ipublish.com.

W A Time Warner Company

Printed in the United States of America
First Printing: October 2001
10 9 8 7 6 5 4 3 2 1

Library of Congress Cataloging-in-Publication Data
Brown, Jack, Ph.D.
    Don't touch that doorknob! : how germs can zap you, and how you can zap back / Jack Brown.
        p.cm.
    Includes bibliographical references and index.
    ISBN 0-446-67634-9
    1.   Microbiology—Popular works. 2. Sanitary microbiology—Popular works. 3. Medical microbiology—Popular works. I. Title.

    QR56 .B68 2001
    616'.01—dc21   00-068599

Book design and text composition by Ellen Gleeson
Cover design by Nina Poliseno
Cover photo by Don Penny

To Mary Ellen, who is good for my heart

Author's Note

The program described in this book is not intended to be a substitute for medical care and advice. You are advised to consult your health-care professional with regard to matters relating to your health, including matters that may require diagnosis or medical attention. In particular, if you are pregnant or have any other special condition requiring medical attention, you should consult regularly with your physician.

The information provided in this book is based on sources that the author believes to be reliable. All such information is current as of August 2000.

Contents

Contents

Don't Touch That Doorknob!

Introduction

Have you ever found yourself in a crowded elevator and wished you were covered in plastic? Or, better yet, that others were? When you're waiting for your groceries to be checked out and the person in front of you sneezes, have you been tempted to drop to the floor and yell, "Incoming!" After a handshake-filled cocktail party, have you ever wondered how long your antibacterial soap lasts? If so, you are like many other folks these days who are concerned about *GERMS!* While the fears may be obvious, the facts are not.

What is a germ, anyway? Is it a bacterium, a virus, a fungus, or perhaps all three? And which one caused that nasty flu you had last winter? And where did you "catch" it? Was the germ passed on through the simple act of shaking someone's hand? Did it ride along in your pocket, cling to your clothing, stick to your shoes, even withstand a wash? Or did you pick it up making dinner in the kitchen or from the sofa while watching TV? Or was your illness due to the combined effects of numerous germs, in all areas of your life?

These important questions and others are a natural reaction to the risks we face from organisms that can cause illness, infection, disease, and sometimes death. No one can be immune to every disease; therefore we all have to learn to live with such microbial tormentors and invaders.

1

The marketplace has responded to our fear of germs with every sort of weaponry to fight them in our homes and on our bodies. There are bathroom foams laced with germ-killing substances, baby rattles impregnated with antibacterial agents, chemical-laden sponges to rid surfaces of the majority of tiny life—you name it, it is out there. Tightly sealed, gleamingly presented, and abundantly advertised, these germ-fighting weapons line the shelves, calming us with their perceived power over the tiny critters with big Latin names. We apparently have a war on our hands, and manufacturers promise that we are equipped with the weapons we need to win. What we may not really understand is why we are in this war in the first place or what the enemies are. Therefore, this book is designed to be a source of common-sense information about both good and bad germs and their impact on all facets of our daily lives.

No amount of information will ever allow us to feel completely comfortable with germs. However, the good news is that only a percentage of these germs is truly harmful and the rest, believe it or not, are actually helpful. While we do not wish to become complacent about the real dangers and risks of infectious disease, we do not want to spend every waking moment paranoid about catching the latest cold that's going around. The intent of this book is to provide a common-sense guide about how to live with the germs all around us. In order to develop this "sense," we need to understand what a germ truly is and where it lurks in our lives. The ensuing chapters will describe certain germs specifically, and will address our interactions with them relative to where we spend our time: with ourselves by living in our skin, in our home and living spaces, in our community, and in our travels.

The term *germ* comes from a derivation of the Latin word for *sprout* and is used collectively to describe all manner of microorganisms. In the first few chapters we will discuss bacteria, viruses, and fungi in substantially more detail. Don't worry, you won't be asked to wade through the complete, unabridged dictionary of all the billions of microorganisms on the face of the planet. Instead we will simply take a look at the more common features associated with bacteria and viruses, with descriptions of a few fungi and maybe even a protozoan or two thrown in for good measure. But if you are dying to know about the bacteria in your cheese or the mold in your shower, skip ahead to the pertinent chapters.

A Brief History of Germs

While technology and research have made it obvious that infectious diseases are caused by microorganisms, this was not the case as recently as the 1860s. Even before true causes of disease were known, there was enough fear and recognition of such symptoms that prudent steps were taken by various populations to prevent the spread of whatever plague was upon them. As far back as the pharaohs of Egypt, we have seen evidence from carvings and paintings that "polio" was as deadly 4,000 years ago as it can be in some parts of the world today. We know from other writings and descriptions that leprosy clearly existed then, as it does now.

The ancient writings of Thucydides, a historian who lived in Greece around 430 B.C., describe what appears to be a plague epidemic within the city. Thucydides even related in some detail how people who were survivors of similar epidemics were specifically selected to care for the sick and dying, since the survivors appeared to be unharmed by the disease the second time around. As far back as the 1400s, the Chinese had already developed a method to immunize (the word comes from the Latin *immunis,* meaning "exempt") individuals to prevent the disease we now know as smallpox. Later, because of the exchange of information that occurred along trade routes to China from Turkey, the Turks used this same form of immunization to protect folks from the ravages of this disease. So, while many cultures throughout history may not have known the exact cause of various diseases, there is historical evidence to show that there was great effort to fight them.

Before the invention of the microscope, the general belief was that if you could not see it, it did not exist. Nobody really understood how sickness could begin and spread among people; even though plagues of different sorts frequently led to many deaths among local populations. Although the Italian physician Girolamo Fracastoro suggested sometime around 1546 that some diseases were caused by invisible organisms, most people related the terrible afflictions to supernatural elements such as witches, the devil, and evil spirits. The "Black Death" that ravaged Europe in the Middle Ages is estimated to have killed more than 25 percent of the population of Europe at the time. Attributed to evil spirits, no one knew that fleas infected with a microorganism known as *Yersinia pestis* were spreading the Death, or bubonic plague as it is now officially known. For more than 1,500 years the plague spread unabated, even after the cause had been determined. As recently as the beginning of the twentieth century, almost 10 million people died of the plague over about a twenty-year period in India.

Hardly anyone before the nineteenth century, including scientists, had any inkling that there might be life-forms smaller than the eye could see, let alone cause such human suffering. Many believed that under the proper conditions life could spring into existence spontaneously in response to some mysterious "life force." Almost everyone talked knowledgeably about this "life force"; however, if one looks for a detailed description of this phenomenon, there are few available.

Until Antoni van Leeuwenhoek's research in the 1670s, no one had seen microorganisms as tiny as a bacterium, much less described them. Leeuwenhoek observed with his own version of a microscope (Galileo was likely the first microscope maker) little critters he named "animalcules." From his detailed descriptions of his find, he had clearly seen bacteria. Even as the years passed with accumulated evidence that life too small to see with the naked eye existed, the belief in spontaneous generation persisted, and was considered to be the cause of disease.

In 1861 Louis Pasteur, through a series of wonderfully designed yet simple experiments, finally convinced the majority of science types that the "life force" theory not only had some holes in it, but was empty to begin with. He proved in a simple experiment that microorganisms did not arise spontaneously "out of thin air" from mysterious forces but instead were already present in the air, on surfaces, and in the water.

Pasteur's procedure involved small hand-blown glass flasks designed with a long, open-ended swan-shaped neck. Because of the ingenious design, unless a person purposefully blew hard into the neck's open end, matter could not easily enter the flask contents. Instead, these particles, which included many microorganisms, settled harmlessly into the bend. Thus, the flask existed without any kind of physical barrier between the environment and the flask's contents, while still allowing the contents to be exposed directly to the "force" thought responsible for the generation of life.

Since scientists knew that heat from a fire could kill living creatures, Pasteur reasoned that if he used heat to kill any microorganisms already present in the flask and broth, the broth should remain clear even though directly exposed to the life force. Consequently, Pasteur flamed the neck of each flask, poured a nutrient-rich broth into the flasks, and brought the broth to a boil, letting it boil for a time. Then Pasteur simply left the flasks exposed to the air in a room. Days, weeks, and months passed, yet not one bit of evidence of "life" appeared inside any of the flasks and the broth remained absolutely clear.

Pasteur then selected some of the flasks at random and tilted the liquid into the bend of the neck—where he hoped the dust and germs were trapped—and allowed the liquid to flow back into the container. Within a few hours the broth inside the flasks turned cloudy and gradually became filled with material, evidence that something was alive and growing inside.

6

Later experiments showed the solid matter consisted of bacteria. This information not only rid the world of the life-force theory, but it also established a methodology of heat treatment to render liquids free of live microorganisms and for rendering foods sterile.

Around this same time, an association between such microscopic life and disease also began to rise. That a fungus could cause a disease in plants was fairly well established by 1845. Such a microorganism proved to be the cause of the Great Potato Blight of Ireland. A physician named Joseph Lister also established a link between microorganisms and disease when, in 1867, he published a simple but highly effective method to prevent infection, or sepsis, in hospitals. At that time physicians did any number of procedures and, consequently, might go directly from performing a surgical procedure to assisting a mother in childbirth. These events would normally occur without hand-washing or a change of clothing between patient contacts. Lister, a well-read person, believed that he could have something unseen on his person that could cause disease in his patients. He found that if he used phenol (carbolic acid) to cleanse his hands between examinations or procedures and to soak his surgical instruments before use, he could prevent sepsis in his patients. This one simple procedure saved countless lives in Lister's day, and it was the basis for the procedures required for maintaining safe conditions in hospitals today.

About ten years after Lister published his work, Robert Koch, a contemporary of Pasteur, established that the disease known as anthrax was caused by a bacterium (*Bacillus anthracis*). In order to establish the connection,

Koch created a procedure to follow when one attempts to associate a given disease with a suspected culprit; which in 1884 became collectively known as Koch's Postulates. These rules require that a microorganism can be isolated from a diseased individual, that pure cultures of this organism can be established, and that a susceptible experimental host, when inoculated with this microorganism, gets the same disease as the original individual. The rules do not stop here. The same organism must again be isolated, but this time from the experimental host, and again given to an additional experimental, susceptible host. The second experimental individual must also get the same disease as the originally ill individual. If all of these conditions are met, the microorganism will be identified as the causative agent of the disease.

While for obvious ethical reasons healthy humans are not used today as experimental susceptible hosts, the history of microbiology and medicine includes many examples of brave individuals who risked their own health as volunteers or as scientists to apply Koch's Postulates. A recent groundbreaking example of such a person is Dr. Barry Marshall, whose inoculation of himself with the bacterium *Helicobacter pylori* established the first step in identifying this bacterium as the causative agent of gastric ulcer disease in humans.

As time passed, more and more information about the association between illnesses and microorganisms became common knowledge. Consequently, instead of a comfortable awareness of the many good things about bacteria, such as their use in the digestive process of the large intestine, most people became fearful of these organisms. Then, when viruses entered the picture in the early 1900s through their scientific identification as the causative agent of a kind of cancer in chickens (by American pathologist Francis Rous) and the easily identifiable affliction poliomyelitis (through the work of Karl Landsteiner), originally known as infantile paralysis, there was yet another group of much smaller enemies to worry about.

Fifty or so years ago, the biggest concern of a parent was probably the danger that his or her child might face from some infectious disease. People were careful to look for any signs of "pneumonia" in their infants or toddlers. Rural kids were sternly warned by their moms, "Don't step on any rusty nails or you might get blood poisoning." Anyone who complained of a sore throat was questioned incessantly and carefully examined for "strep." The presence of scarlet fever brought anxiety running instead of Rhett Butler. And as recently as forty years ago there was probably not a parent in the United States who did not fear that his or her child might "catch polio" while swimming during the summer. As a consequence, there were far fewer fun-filled gatherings of crowds of youngsters yelling and splashing in pools on their vacations. These fears were well founded, but there was also general acceptance in those years that risks of infection from germs were always present. One simply hoped for the best and avoided obvious dangers.

The anxiety of childhood infection began to shift somewhat with the appearance of penicillin, the "wonder drug" of the twentieth century. Beginning with the widespread availability of this antibiotic during the 1940s, great strides continued to be made by the scientific and medical communities in regard to the fight against infectious agents. Use of different and improved antibiotics and the development of vaccines began to make a dent in people's fears. The concerns about polio, "lockjaw," whooping cough, and the like began to fade somewhat as these apparent victories over the scourges of humankind began to mount. So why worry any longer about pneumonia, or "strep," or tetanus, or pretty much any kind of bacterial infection? We could easily cure it with the proper antibiotic. Why worry about some virus thing? All one needs to do to cure oneself is swallow a few pills a couple of times a week.

Now, however, with the appearance of things like HIV, the West Nile virus, and *E. coli*, fear is on the rise again. Outbreaks of terrible viral diseases, such as those caused by the *Ebola* virus family, the increase in resistance to antibiotics by various harmful bacteria (i.e., supergerms), and the suspected use of germ warfare during the Gulf War have heightened awareness. Worst-case-scenario thrillers and medical mumbo-jumbo movies have just made the panic worse. Therefore, it is very hard not to be hypervigilant about the situation.

How and whom do we fight? There are no simple solutions, nor is there one easy procedure that will always kill the bad germs and save the good germs—at least not yet. What, then, are we to do? Perhaps the best plan is to identify our real enemies, determine our day-to-day risk of an encounter with these thugs, and just see what we can do to increase the numbers of the good guys. All in all, perhaps we can find a way to live with the germs around us.

Chapter One

Microorganisms–
The Large World of Small Life

Welcome to the large world of small life—the world of microorganisms. This chapter will introduce you to many of the little critters that will be discussed specifically in later chapters. Please keep in mind that although there are some rogues among them, the overwhelming number of germs are truly amazing and surprisingly helpful to us.

What is considered a microorganism?

This microorganic world includes such things as bacteria, viruses, fungi, algae, and protozoa. Because they are so tiny and are commonly invisible to the naked eye, the field that studies these organisms is named microbiology. To provide some perspective on just how small "tiny" is, the smallest object the human eye can see is 200 millionths of a meter in size. For comparison, the dot atop the following "i" is about 2 1/2 times bigger than the smallest particle visible to the human eye. Individual cells, including those of bacteria, for example, are much, much smaller, maybe 50 to 100 times smaller. Viruses are even tinier. At least 50 million of the virus that causes polio can fit into an average-size human cell—a cell that is about 50 times smaller than the smallest dot visible to the human eye. Twenty-five thousand bacteria can be lined up end to end on a one-inch-long blade of grass—and that is not even taking into account the algae, fungi, and protozoa that can also exist in the same location. So if your eye can't spot the darn thing without help from a microscope, take my word for it: that thing is really, really small.

Are there many of these microorganisms on the earth?

Before the first microscope was invented, the only things thought to exist were those that could actually be seen. I expect people of years ago would be astonished to know that, relative to all of the living organisms that can be seen on this earth, the ones that cannot be seen are far greater in number.

Although we do not find fungi, algae, or protozoa in the news very much (when was the last time you saw an article with "protozoa" in the title?), that is not the case when it comes to bacteria and viruses. We may hear or read about these particular bugs almost every day. When we do, the news is usually about some disease, so we quite naturally tend to be more frightened of these organisms.

While I grant you that there aren't many nice things to say about viruses, when it comes to bacteria, this is not the case. While some bacteria can be vicious, the vast majority is extremely good for us. Bacteria are the most abundant living things on our planet. They can be found on the highest mountaintop, inside the hardest rocks, miles below the surface in ancient ice of Antarctica, and in the deepest depths of the ocean around volcanic vents. Their ability to adapt and survive is absolutely amazing. Most important, without them, life as we know it—not just you and me, but all life— would not exist on this earth.

> Bacteria represent at least 5,000 different species. It is estimated that only half are actually identified.

While there are scads of bacteria around, there are many more different identified species of protozoa, algae, and fungi. Most are not harmful to humans but have the ability to be. For example, some single-cell algae may be dangerous because of poisonous substances they can release into the water, such as those that form what we call a "red tide." These toxic substances can be concentrated within the tissues of shellfish and can be toxic if eaten. Even accidentally ingesting a bunch of these algae can be harmful, so avoid swimming if a red tide is present.

The organisms known as plankton are algae, too. Their abundant floating presence along the oceans of the earth not only provides food for marine life but is believed to be the source of about half of the oxygen we breathe—most of the balance is thought to be provided by the many bacteria that live in the ocean. (Yes, we do get some oxygen from plants, too.)

Are there some microorganisms that you can see or touch?

The enormous variability among these germs includes remarkable differences in size, shape, function, and capacities to live in strange places. Their size can fool you; some forms of these microorganisms are actually very large. Ocean-dwelling kelp and seaweed, made up of lots of individual algae cells connected to one another, can be taller than the tallest tree on land and have appendages a person could easily mistake for leaves.

And what about those mushrooms that sometimes spring up like little umbrellas on the forest floor? Those mushrooms aren't funny-looking individuals; they are actually part of a bigger living organism growing just underneath the soil's surface. Scientists discovered one enormous fungus that spreads over 2 1/2 acres beneath the soil—that's larger than two football fields—and is thought to be between 1,000 and 1,500 years old. Beyond such rare size exceptions, the majority is truly tiny.

Are microorganisms actually alive?

Explaining the meaning of life in relation to germs can sometimes be frustrating. Researchers debate this issue fairly frequently. Here is the tried-and-true, hard-line scientific definition: Life is the ability to reproduce, the ability to exist independently as a complete organism, and possession of all of the biochemical processes that allow reproduction and independent existence to occur. Similar to higher life-forms like humans, when microorganisms reproduce, all of the necessary genetic information is continuously passed from one generation to the next. However, how well the information is accurately passed along determines the ability to exist as individuals.

The single exception to this definition of life involves viruses. The jury is still out as to whether viruses are actually alive. Viruses reproduce—prolifically, in fact—and can exist as individual members of different groups. Genetic material is copied and passed along from generation to generation. So why aren't viruses considered to be alive? A virus can neither reproduce nor survive as a completely independent thing: A virus must be inside a living cell and depends upon the cell's machinery in order to produce more of its kind. Furthermore, the virus cannot remain active (functional) for very long outside a living cell. Some people think these organisms are a form of pseudo-life or partial life. For our purposes, we will consider a virus to be a biologically functional little package of genetic material, but not a living thing.

All of the other tiny organisms we'll discuss will be treated as different forms of life. Although bacteria and viruses will be the primary focus of our environmental journey, we will also talk about some of the interesting and sometimes harmful aspects of certain algae, fungi, and protozoa.

In Summary

- *Germ* is the term commonly used to describe any microorganism.
- If it is too tiny to be seen without the aid of a microscope, it is a microorganism.

- Microorganisms include such things as bacteria, viruses, fungi, algae, and protozoa.
- Bacteria, viruses, protozoa, and the single-cell forms of algae and fungi are, with only one or two exceptions, invisible to the human eye.
- Bacteria represent the most abundant form of life on the planet.
- Except for viruses, all microorganisms are considered to be living.
- Human life would not exist without bacteria.

Chapter Two

Bacteria–They're Everywhere! They're Everywhere!

Bacteria exist everywhere on this planet: Both the ocean and soil are absolutely loaded with them. So are human beings. Most bacteria spend their lives as a single cell, but, like most of us, they are surrounded by neighbors. Many different species exist together in complex populations on just about any surface, whether in the wild reaches of your yard or on your skin. In a sense, we are constantly awash in a virtual sea of bacteria from the time we are born until the time we leave this earth.

> More than 200 different species of bacteria are estimated to live around a single tooth!

Under normal conditions bacteria help us, but bacterial bad behavior is what you'll read about in the headlines.

What does a bacterium look like?

Bacteria come in a myriad of different shapes and sizes—some are round, some are rod-like, and some are even square. But no matter the shape, the most common form is unicellular, or consisting of a single cell. They can exist either individually (which is relatively uncommon) or as a dependent group of individual cells in colonies. These colonies often interconnect with other colonies to form their own self-sufficient ecosystems. For example, the waste products from one bacterial community can provide food for a different group. Because of the different colors of substances bacteria may produce, given enough time, these colored layers of little communities, each consisting of millions and millions of cells, will appear in something as simple as a jar filled with pond mud. Individual colonies of bacteria growing on a petri plate are also visible without the aid of a microscope. Sometimes colored and sometimes not, the aggregate of millions of cells that arise from a single cell usually looks like a little raised, opaque dot on a smooth surface.

How long can a bacterium live?

Many bacteria have a life span as short as twenty minutes prior to dividing into two new cells. But if the food runs out, they will die. Others suspend all of their biologic processes when food is scarce; in this state of suspended animation they can last for weeks without apparent harm. Still others can assume a different form, known as a spore, and exist with no apparent life activity for many years. Scientists have found and revived spores more than 9,000 years old.

For many of these microorganisms, the lack of a complete diet isn't necessarily a problem: Bacteria are able to metabolize and derive nutrients and energy from just about any organic or inorganic substance, from starch compounds and sugars to iron and sulfur. Some bacteria can even make their own food from sunlight, using a process known as photosynthesis. Other bacteria, such as the microbes that reside in your digestive system, simply munch on the food you have already digested.

Like children, bacteria apparently thrive with good nutrition, and they reproduce continuously when sufficient food is available. This particular property is useful to keep in mind when we talk about food safety and bacterial contamination in later chapters.

How do bacteria reproduce?

Bacteria reproduce by a method called binary fission, or division by twos. Basically, the cell gets bigger and bigger until it reaches about twice the normal size, duplicates the genetic material (a single chromosome), and then divides in half, with the contents split between the two new cells. The result is two identical cells from one, each containing a single

> If a cell divided every twenty minutes, it would take less than seven hours for only *one* bacterial cell to become more than *one million* identical cells.

chromosome that has all of the information needed for the life of that cell. The two new cells can reproduce, and so on, giving quick rise to a group, called a colony, of millions of identical cells. This ability to reproduce in a blink of an eye can make dangerous bacteria very dangerous. Without assistance our bodies cannot cope with such an onslaught. But this same property can make good bacteria very good: Give them half a chance and they will scrub the environment clean of toxic substances.

Do we depend on bacteria for anything?

Two of the many things bacteria do for humans are to produce certain necessary vitamins and to help digest our food. But that is not all. One of the bacteria found both in the soil and in the dust—the genus *Streptomyces*—provides the majority of antibiotics used to cure bacterial infections.

Bacteria not only make useful drugs and enzymes but serve a greater purpose as well. Bacteria in the soil such as *Rhizobium* convert nitrogen, which is necessary for all life, into a form usable by most living organisms. When a living thing dies, other bacteria change the nitrogen back to nitrogen gas, allowing the gas to re-enter the atmosphere. This necessary cycle occurs every

Streptomyces, the family of bacteria that structurally resemble some fungi, are extremely useful. The majority of antibiotics that are used for human and veterinary medicine, such as tetracycline and erythromycin, come from these germs. They are also the source of other useful substances, some of which kill parasites, some of which kill weeds, and some that suppress the immune system (for people getting an organ transplant, for example). These bacteria provide enzymes for the food industry, as well.

second of every day throughout the entire world, thanks to bacteria.

Do "good" bacteria help to keep the bad germs away?

The mass of non-pathogenic bacteria and other organisms that live happily within us often serve as indirect protectors. When a pathogen enters our body, there is a potential for that organism to cause an infection. But because of the enormous competition for nutrients and the lack of available space to attach to our exposed tissue, most pathogens die rather quickly. Even if they do survive, having to fight for space and nutrients with other germs will help insure that they do not increase to a harmful level.

What makes bacteria dangerous?

When we are trying to decide whether bacteria are helpful or harmful, there are two important things to consider: their number and what they produce. Except under very unusual circumstances, one little bacterium acting alone does not have the strength either to harm or to help us. But once there are thousands or millions of them, things can change in a hurry. Depending upon the type of bacteria present, a large number can be either a danger or an asset. For example, when the *Exxon Valdez* struck a reef in Alaska's Prince William Sound in 1989, oil-eating bacteria were able to increase quickly in number and help clean the ocean and beaches.

The ability to increase rapidly in number is an amazing characteristic of bacteria (and, as we will find out in

21

the next chapter, it is even more amazing in viruses.) Consider this calculation: If a bacterium divides every twenty minutes (a common feat for this little critter) and none of the cells die, within approximately forty-three hours there would be enough to fill the entire volume of the earth. I grant you, it is not a pretty thought, but it makes a point.

One reason we are not wading through bacteria is because most of the cells die. Bacteria require a lot of energy simply to stay alive. With the constant internal demands of cell division and competition for food and water, it is easy to understand why only the fittest cells survive.

Sometimes the total number of bacteria is less important than what the bugs produce. Some of these disease-causing (pathogenic) bacteria don't even have to be present to cause terrible problems. *Clostridium botulinum* can cause an infection and also produce dangerous toxins that can cause paralysis and, ultimately, death. However, *C. botulinum* doesn't actually need to infect you to hurt you: The toxin produced by this bacterium remains lethal in improperly canned food long after the bacterium itself has died.

Where are the bacteria hiding?

Unlike the exposed surfaces of our bodies, which teem with different microorganisms, the inside of our bodies does not normally play host to as many living organisms. An exception is the intestines, which harbor thousands of bacteria that are necessary for us to remain healthy.

However, bacteria can gain entry to regions not usually accessible to them through an open wound or if organisms are pushed into a normally sterile region. For example, a urinary tract infection is caused when *E. coli* is pushed into the urethra (the tube leading from the bladder) through improper wiping and begins to grow.

How can all of this information be of use?

The more we understand about bacteria, the easier it is to help them help us, and to keep them from harming us. For example, we have learned and are still learning how to fight harmful bacteria by attacking them in places where they are vulnerable. We can use that same knowledge to provide the right conditions to help increase the number of helpful bacteria in a given location. As we will see in later chapters, this kind of information gives us a handle on how to live with these bugs, both the good and the bad among them.

In Summary

- Outside of a few exceptions, bacterial cells are too small to see without a microscope.
- There are lots of different kinds of bacteria, with the majority being helpful to humans.
- When there are enough nutrients, bacteria reproduce like mad.
- Bacteria are all around us, and all life on earth depends upon their existence.

Chapter Three

Viruses–The Ultimate Internal Alien

First let's talk about what a virus is *not*. A virus is not a bacterium, nor is it an independently living organism. A virus can neither survive for very long nor replicate without being inside a living cell. Antibiotics do not harm viruses; they are designed to kill bacteria. Certain antiviral drugs have worked with limited success, but because of the wide variety of viruses, there aren't many of these drugs available. In almost all cases of a viral infection, we depend on our own immune response to fight it off and take medicine just to ease the symptoms of the infection.

Well then, what is a virus?

Similar to a living organism, a virus has some fundamental genetic information, either DNA or RNA, which allows it to replicate. When the virus replicates, it is active. When it does not, it is considered inactive. Thus, a virus is not strictly alive, nor is it strictly dead.

A virus is very, very small relative to the size of a living cell and can be viewed only with an electron microscope. The biggest virus known is fifty- to one-hundred-fold smaller than the smallest bacterium. As an example, the head of a straight pin could hold about 50 million of the viruses that cause the common cold. While their size makes them too small to replicate on their own, viruses have evolved to use the mechanism of a host cell to replicate.

How does a virus survive?

A virus is not only an accomplished thief, it is also an equally successful freeloader. A virus uses a cell's machinery, enzymes, and, in some cases, genetic material to generate virus parts—all at the expense of the cell. The cell is also used as a breeding ground for hundreds, thousands, and sometimes millions of new, mature, infectious viruses that can leave the cell to infect other cells. After one takes hold, it can take less than thirty minutes for more than 100 viruses to appear inside that cell.

How exactly does a virus infect a host cell?

Once a virus comes across a potential host cell, it immediately attaches itself to the cell. Then the virus, fusing itself with the outside of the cell's membrane (in the case of an animal virus) or cell wall (in the case of a bacterial virus), will either enter the cell as a complete entity (in the animal virus) or will act like a hypodermic needle and inject its genetic material inside the cell (in the bacterial virus). If the virus uses DNA for its genetic material, this DNA can remain in the host cell's cytoplasm, or enter the nucleus (in a eukaryotic cell) or can even be incorporated into the original DNA of the host cell in order to be replicated. If the virus uses RNA for its genetic material, the RNA can be either immediately used to produce viral proteins and then replicated or replicated first. Regardless of the kind of genetic material, or genome (DNA or RNA), there will eventually be many copies of that viral genome and ultimately the cell will be transformed into a factory for replicating the complete virus. For example, the poliomyelitis virus, which causes polio, may have over 1 million copies of its basic genetic information (RNA) inside a single infected human intestinal cell.

As the virus multiplies within the cell, new viruses escape from inside by either blowing the cell apart or squeezing out of the cell and taking some membranes with them as they leave. In both instances the cell eventually dies from the damage. But, strangely, infection by a virus does not always cause disease. For example, about 95 percent of adults are infected with the latent form of the Epstein-Barr virus (EBV), but only a small percentage of those infected get the disease mononucleosis, which is caused by EBV.

Viruses are certainly fascinating creatures; if you would like to learn more about them, one Web site that provides interesting, easy-to-understand information is Hidden Killers: Virus Basics at http://library.thinkquest.org.

What can a virus infect?

Every living thing—plants, animals, bacteria—whether many-celled or single-celled, can be infected with a virus specific for the organism. Usually, a particular virus will have only one target. There are, of course, exceptions to the one-virus-one-target rule: Influenza virus Type A can infect pigs, birds, and humans; the West Nile virus can infect birds, horses, and humans; and the rabies virus can infect humans as well as many other warm-blooded animals.

What does a virus look like?

Although they may have similar features, viruses on the whole look very different from each other, ranging in appearance from round to worm-like to angular. If you want to see different microorganisms, visit Dr. Linda Stannard's Web site at www.uct.ac.za/depts/mmi/stannard/linda.html.

Why do viruses exist?

Viruses exist only to make more viruses. With the possible exception of those that target antibiotic-resistant bacteria, there is no evidence that viruses do humans any good at all.

Why are viruses so harmful?

Viruses are dangerous because their replication inside the cell leads to the death of that cell. Viruses can multiply in number and spread throughout an organism very quickly, essentially overwhelming any prevention system the organism might have. Depending on the strength of the virus and the quality and speed of our immune response against it, the effects of infection by one virus can range from brief discomfort to death.

Why do antibiotics not work against viruses?

Antibiotics are designed to fight bacteria, which have a different structure than viruses. Bacteria have self-sufficient prokaryotic systems that are very different from the systems of humans and so can be attacked without significant risk to the human body. However, viruses replicate using human cells as their host. Therefore, any medicine we design to harm a virus might harm us by hurting the cells the virus inhabits. Scientists who design antiviral medicine must target aspects of the virus that do not affect humans.

However, the influenza viruses can cause such damage to the airways and lungs that a person can become particularly vulnerable to a subsequent bacterial infection of the lungs. That is why an antibiotic may be prescribed as a preventative measure against an additional infection caused by bacteria, such as bacterial pneumonia. The danger of bacterial pneumonia as a serious complication of the flu is further discussed in Chapter Seven.

There are a few drugs that are useful against certain viruses: amantadine, rimantadine, zanamivir, and oseltamivir. Amantadine (approved in 1966) and rimantadine (approved in 1993) are effective against influenza virus Type A, and only so if taken within forty-eight hours of infection. These drugs interfere with the ability of the virus to make more viruses. Zanamivir and oseltamivir are two newer drugs (approved in 1999) that are effective against both Type A and B of the influenza virus.

They interfere with the activity of one of the enzymes (neuraminidase) necessary for these different strains of influenza virus to infect cells. A very recently developed drug (AG7088) against rhinovirus, the virus that causes the common cold, was the object of a Phase II clinical trial initiated in 1999. Also, you may be familiar with the drug named acyclovir that is used to inhibit the replication of herpes virus, and with AZT and HIV protease inhibitors that are used to inhibit the replication of HIV.

Do viruses change?

Sometimes when a virus replicates, mutations can occur in its genetic material that may cause it no longer to be functional or infectious. However, some mutations may just change the way the virus looks, which may also be dangerous to us. Our immune system recognizes molecular shapes, and if the shapes change, a new response must be generated in order to be effective soon enough to prevent harm. These changes in a virus's appearance are what lead to brand-new strains of the virus. The influenza virus can do this; consequently, there are several different strains of this virus identified each year that make up the vaccine against the flu.

Is there anything that can stop the spread of a virus in our body?

If a virus infects one or more cells in our body, these cells will release protein substances called interferons. These proteins enable adjacent cells to become more resistant to infection by the virus. Sometimes the interferons are not enough to prevent the spread of the virus and we begin to feel sick. Our immune system then responds by killing the virus on the outside of the cells and the infected cells, too. Since a virus requires a living cell in order to be able to survive and multiply, killing the infected cells prevents the spread of the virus. If the virus hasn't harmed one of our body's vital functions, it will be completely removed by the immune system, and, if we are otherwise healthy, we should get over the illness.

Other viruses, such as human immunodeficiency virus (HIV), are not so easy to kill. HIV infects the very cells of the immune system that are necessary for our ability to fight not only HIV, but also all other viral and bacterial infections. So, although HIV does not itself directly cause the condition known as AIDS, it causes the eventual death of immune cells, which allows other infections to run rampant.

As this chapter's subhead says, a virus is indeed the ultimate internal alien. Time now to go forward and leave the very tiny world of viruses and head for algae, fungi, and protozoa.

In Summary

- A virus is not a bacterium.
- A virus cannot reproduce outside of a living cell.
- Every living thing has a specific virus that can infect it.
- Scientists estimate that, outside of a living cell, a virus can last for days at the most.
- Some viruses are deadly, some are not.

- Antivirals, not antibiotics, kill viruses.
- Viruses cause many different diseases, including the common cold, flu, and pneumonia, as well as diseases such as measles, mumps, and encephalitis (infection of the brain).

Chapter Four

Algae, Fungi, and Protozoa– Get to Know Them

Almost everyone is familiar with both algae and fungi in one form or another, usually as scum on a pond or toadstools in the grass. But protozoa are a lot less familiar. Algae and fungi usually do us a world of good by making oxygen, getting rid of dead matter, and serving as the source of many potent antibiotics. But anyone who has ever been sickened by eating toxin-loaded shellfish or had a yeast infection or "athlete's foot" knows that these groups have their bad side, too. Protozoa, on the other hand, do not necessarily do us any obvious good but play an important role in the earth's chain of life. Their bad guys are just as bad, though. One type of protozoa, *Entamoeba histolytica,* for example, can contaminate the water of lakes, streams, and rivers and, when ingested, can lead to the severe acute gastrointestinal disease known as amoebic dysentery.

Algae, fungi, and protozoa have one very important feature in common with human cells: the presence of a nucleus. Having a nucleus means these cells possess operating systems similar to our own cells'. Similarities, such as the systems that involve DNA and RNA usage, mean that the cellular machinery of algae, fungi, and protozoa are closely related to human cellular machinery and therefore are more difficult to target for harm. Consequently, if we happen to become infected with one of them, it becomes more difficult to kill them without hurting ourselves.

What are algae?

Algae love water. Salt or fresh, it doesn't matter—water is where you will find them. They live in lakes, oceans, and even inside other organisms, such as coral (they produce food for the coral). Algae can form on damp walls or within moist soil, but if it is dry they will die. Like plants, most algae make their own food through photosynthesis. Some algae, however, can't use the sun for energy to make their food; they do not have chlorophyll, so they use the energy of living cells. It is within this limited group of algae that the single known group of infectious algae is found: three members of the genus *Prototheca*.

Some members of the unicellular algae, *Prototheca*, are becoming more recognized as a possible source of human infection. Found all over the place in water (lakes and ponds) and moist soil, these germs most commonly infect us via small wounds in the feet or hands. The skin disease caused by this organism is known as protothecosis. Infection by these organisms is to date extremely rare—only about sixty or so cases have been reported throughout the world (most of these within the southeastern United States)—but the fact that reports are appearing is an indication that a new pathogen may be emerging. So far, most of these infections have appeared in individuals whose immune system is weakened for one reason or another (those with diabetes, those who are organ-transplant recipients, and persons receiving chemotherapy). These organisms are thought to be opportunistic pathogens: They do not usually infect a healthy individual and can gain a foothold only when something else is wrong.

Most algae exist as single cells but some species, such as kelp and seaweed, are many-celled and can become large plant-like structures. While human infection is rare, the group of algae known as dinoflagellates are dangerous because they release poisons. There are several different combinations of poisons that may be involved. There are neurotoxins known as NSPs (neurotoxin shellfish poisons) that can cause severe distress. Other toxins, ASPs (amnesic shellfish poisons), can cause short-term memory loss if enough is ingested. Probably the worst of the lot are PSPs (paralytic shellfish poisons), which can kill us. These dangerous substances can be absorbed and concentrated in certain edible shellfish. Whenever the conditions such as temperature and food supply are ideal, dinoflagellates can greatly increase in number and cover large areas of the water, fresh or salt. These visible accumulations are known as an algal "bloom" or "red tide." If fish or shellfish feed in the area, they can accumulate the toxins; consequently if someone eats the contaminated fish, they will be contaminated as well. Unfortunately, cooking the shellfish has little effect on these toxins—they remain dangerous.

If you've read the book or seen the movie *The Perfect Storm,* you will recognize the setting of Georges Bank, a long-existing commercial fishing area about 100 miles

From the Washington State Department of Health: "The Biotoxin Program monitors levels of Paralytic Shellfish Poison (PSP), formerly referred to as 'red tide,' and Amnesic Shellfish Poison (ASP or domoic acid) in molluscan shellfish. A PSP Hotline lists beaches that are closed to recreational harvest due to significant levels of biotoxins." This Health Department closed several areas in 2000 to recreational clam, oyster, and mussel harvest due to shellfish toxins.

east of Cape Cod, Massachusetts. This is the same location where, back in 1990, the crew of a commercial fishing boat almost died from respiratory paralysis after steaming and eating toxin-contaminated shellfish they found in their nets. The source of the toxins was thought to be due to a "bloom" of the dinoflagellate *Alexandrium*. Luckily, the captain of the vessel had sufficient strength to radio the Coast Guard in time to airlift the crew to a hospital on Nantucket Island. All of the ship's crew was saved because of prompt diagnosis and action by the hospital's emergency room personnel. Since certain clams (surf clams) are able to retain the toxin for many years, the U.S. Government (which has jurisdiction over Georges Bank) banned the harvest of these clams in the area.

Are mushrooms the only type of fungi we can eat?

Out of the hundreds of thousands of different species of fungi, the vast majority does not harm humans. The yeast used to make bread rise is actually a single-cell type of fungi (usually *Saccharomyces cerevisiae* or baker's yeast) that can crank out carbon dioxide like crazy as long as there is plenty of sugar for it to eat. When it eats, the breakdown of sugar releases carbon dioxide that bubbles into the dough and provides that fluffy, leavened texture. Yeast cells not only make carbon dioxide but, under conditions where oxygen is not around, they can also make alcohol.

While we recognize many of the good fungi, you are more than likely familiar with at least a few of the bad ones. Some of these things are deadly poisonous. Some are also prone to damaging plants. Remember the potato famine in Ireland: It was a fungus, *Phytophthora infestan,* that killed the potato crops. This infestation ultimately generated a widespread famine throughout the country. As a result, hundreds of thousands of people died during the years 1845–47.

Certainly far less tragic but nonetheless sad is the current condition of our nation's stately elms. A fungus carried by a tree-boring bark beetle is responsible for the fatal condition known as Dutch elm disease. This fungus is spreading insidiously and irrevocably among our elm trees, and there is currently no cure.

What fungi will cause trouble?

Beyond those fungi that harm plant life, about 300 species can cause harm to humans. Certain species of fungal organisms can cause very irritating and uncomfortable respiratory, urogenital, or gastrointestinal infections. For example, the organism *Candida albicans* is the most common culprit responsible for what is most commonly known as a "yeast" infection. Overall, 75 percent of adult women have at least one yeast infection during their lives. And, although the infection is not necessarily dangerous to a healthy woman, it is very irritating and tends to reoccur.

Candida albicans is commonly found to be a normal inhabitant of the mouth, genitals, and skin. Usually, the numbers are low and are held in check by the other normal flora as well as the body's level of acidity. Whenever conditions change, perhaps associated with taking birth control pills or as a result of the menstrual cycle or antibiotic therapy (which can remove competing normal bugs), the yeast cells can become more competitive and can overgrow and replace the other inhabitants. That is when and how a yeast infection occurs. The oral form of this infection is called thrush, which is more common in elderly women due to the lowered saliva production caused by the natural result of aging (saliva inhibits the growth of these organisms). Additionally, medication or antibiotic usage in this population can also sometimes lead to an oral yeast infection. Luckily, effective treatment is available for thrush; there are also topical ointments for treatment of vaginal yeast infections. Drugs such as Diflucan and others can be taken internally to fight both vaginal and oral infections caused by this organism.

Any fungal disease left untreated can be dangerous. But even in otherwise healthy people there are several fungi that can really cause problems. The first, *Blastomyces dermatitidis,* is responsible for the lung disease known as blastomycosis. (You may recognize it as Chicago disease.) Another one is *Coccidioides immitis,* the cause of coccidioidomycosis, which can lead to meningitis and acute pneumonia. This one, also known as valley fever, is probably the worst of the lot and is usually found in the southwestern United States and in the San Joaquin valley in California.

You might also be unlucky enough to be familiar with "athlete's foot," a skin condition caused by the fungus *Trichophyton*. Dermatologists spend a lot of time—and we spend a lot of money—trying to cure ourselves of skin conditions caused by fungi that love to live on and in dead skin, like calluses and toenails. Fingernail and toenail fungal infections are very difficult to treat with pills taken over a short period of time because the infected areas are no longer connected to the bloodstream except right at their growing point. And creams are often not very effective because the dead skin is resistant to the absorption of anything. So about the only way to really get at the infection is to kill the bug as the new fingernail or toenail grows, an expensive treatment that requires taking an internal medication for several months.

Certain fungi can also release harmful toxins. One of these toxins, aflatoxin, when ingested has the strong potential to cause animal and human cells to become cancerous. So avoid eating any food that has become moldy with any mold that is not a normal part of the food-making process (like blue cheese, for example, which utilizes *Penicillium*).

What are my chances of bumping into a protozoan?

The last member of this chapter's triad is the protozoa. Like algae and fungal cells, protozoan cells have a nucleus. So members of the protozoa may have characteristics akin to animals. In fact, the name *protozoan* means "first animal."

These organisms are generally single cells, and most, but not all, of them can move around quite well on their own. They tend to live in wet environments of salt or fresh water and know how to swim. Protozoa can live within cells or tissues of larger creatures and cause no harm. There is even one species that lives inside the gut of a termite, digesting the cellulose the termites have eaten.

Some species of protozoa have outer shell coverings, live in the ocean, and have quite a history. Their fossil deposits that formed some limestone and sandstone, for example, have contributed to the construction of buildings throughout the world. In fact, the ancient pyramids of Egypt are made of limestone that consists mostly of fossilized, shell-type protozoa—that is a lot of protozoa.

Within this big group of living organisms is a small number that can cause diseases in humans, mostly due to untreated water and poor hygiene. Since most protozoa can be found in the water of lakes, streams, and rivers, one obvious problem for humans and animals alike is their possible presence in drinking water. If we ingest one of the varieties that can live within, we are in for some trouble. One problematic characteristic is their capacity to convert to a hard-to-kill form known as a cyst that occurs when environmental conditions aren't favorable, such as when there is a lack of food. The form is reversible, however, and when the environmental restrictions are relieved, the cyst reverts to a vegetative cell. In this form, the organism actively causes us problems, but it is also the form that makes the protozoa vulnerable to treatment.

Two particularly harmful protozoa, *Giardia* and *Cryptosporidium,* may occur in almost any stream or river. Each occurs naturally in the intestines of many wild animals and therefore can be easily spread. Both can cause a diarrheal disease in humans that can be especially harmful to those with weakened immune systems. Other problems various protozoa can cause are sexually transmitted diseases, general kinds of organ infections, or even the disease malaria.

In Summary

- On the whole, algae, fungi, and protozoa are mostly harmless and often helpful, but occasionally they may cause long-lasting illnesses.
- Red tides are caused by poisonous algae called dinoflagellates.
- Some algae produce toxins that we can ingest when we eat shellfish, whether it is raw or cooked.
- Some fungi can cause yeast and other infections.
- Certain protozoa can cause gastrointestinal illness as well as malaria.

Chapter Five

Antibiotic, Antiviral, and Antifungal Agents—Sometimes We Can't Do It on Our Own

While our immune system is a great front-line defense against germs, sometimes it requires a little help. Help is usually provided in the form of an antimicrobial of one kind or another that exploits a germ's weakness. In this chapter we will talk about some of the substances that are used to fight infections.

What is an antimicrobial?

The comprehensive term *antimicrobial,* which means a substance that kills all microorganisms, is finding more common use among scientists as well as the public at large. If you do not think so, just read a few of the labels on household cleaning materials. Many of these products claim to be effective at killing both harmful bacteria and viruses. Of course, dipping a hand in hydrochloric acid would most likely whack any self-respecting bacterium into oblivion, but such a treatment, although antimicrobial in nature, is obviously not the best method. Since household bleach as well as certain prescription drugs are both antimicrobial, let's detail how both work.

What are antibiotics?

The strict scientific definition for an antibiotic is any substance produced by one living microorganism that can kill or inhibit the growth of a different living microorganism. However, the common use of the term refers only to substances that harm bacteria.

Why do we need to take an antibiotic?

As discussed earlier, bacteria can multiply in numbers rapidly if conditions are right. One of the "right" conditions occurs when a bacterium capable of infecting us and causing disease (a pathogen) does just that and begins to multiply. We then have a war on our hands, and the enemy has the initial advantage—in both speed and number. This advantage can ultimately lead to a defeat of our system's defenses. Antibiotics balance the playing field by providing time for the immune system to gear up against the enemy: Antibiotics kill the invaders quickly, greatly reducing their number and keeping the offenders at bay. This action allows our natural defense systems eventually to gain the upper hand and completely defeat the infection. (For more information, see Chapter Seven.)

Where do we get our antibiotics?

Most of the antibiotics we use today are produced from two types of bacteria: *Streptomyces* (the fungi-like bacteria we talked about) and *Bacillus*. The next largest producers are two types of fungi: *Penicillium* and

Cephalosporium. Some antibiotics come from human invention, made from scratch in the laboratory. Others are made by germs but are chemically changed in the laboratory to make them more effective, by increasing potency, making them resistant to stomach acid, or making them more broadly effective against different kinds of bacteria.

How do antibiotics work?

Antibiotics target the vulnerable systems of bacteria, including the cell wall; the internal machinery where proteins are made; the membrane that surrounds a bacterial cell's contents; and the processes necessary for bacteria to maintain their chemically healthy DNA.

All forms of penicillin, vancomycin, and cephalosporin antibiotics block the ability of a bacterium to build a cell wall. Incomplete construction causes this weakened structure to rupture under the chemical stress of a bacterium's life, causing the cell to die.

Other antibiotics such as polymyxin B harm the bacterial plasma membrane. However, our cells have membranes too, so it is dangerous to take these antibiotics internally, though they can be used safely on the skin's surface (topically) for small scratches and abrasions. That's why we see the warning, "For topical use only" on a lot of first-aid creams and ointments.

Antibiotics like streptomycin, erythromycin, and the tetracyclines prevent new proteins from being made by the bacteria, thus killing the cell. The antibiotics that interfere with DNA production are the quinolones and fluroquinolones, which include norfloxacin and ciprofloxacin. This group of antibiotics is particularly effective against bacteria that cause pneumonia, dysentery, and urinary-tract infections.

Can antibiotics hurt me?

Some antibiotics can hurt us, either directly or indirectly. Allergic reaction is a common example, but not everyone is susceptible. If you are allergic to penicillin derivatives, you may also be allergic to any one of the different cephalosporins. If you take an antibiotic and feel flushed or feel "funny" or see a reddish rash anywhere on your body or have shortness of breath—any one or more of these symptoms—call your doctor immediately.

In addition to allergic reactions, some antibiotics can cause other kinds of problems. Antibiotics like streptomycin may damage the eighth cranial nerve. This nerve has two branches: one that involves hearing (the auditory branch) and one that involves balance (the vestibular branch). So, if when taking such an antibiotic you feel dizzy or hear "ringing" in your ears, call your doctor immediately.

Since antibiotics can't determine whether a particular bug is good or bad, any kind of antibiotic therapy can also kill good bacteria, too. We depend on many of these good bugs to help digest our food, so killing them may cause gastrointestinal distress. Eating things like yogurt or drinking buttermilk or "sweet acidophilus" products may help reestablish the necessary bacteria and ease our symptoms.

Are antibiotic-resistant bugs a serious problem?

Dangerous bacteria now exist that are resistant to some of the best antibiotics available. The resistance may be caused through a natural mutation or by acquiring the genetic information from the environment (from other already resistant germs, in particular). The mechanism of resistance may either prevent the entrance of the drug into the bacterium or destroy the drug once it is inside the bacterium. As a consequence, the more indiscriminately antibiotics are used, the greater the chance that a resistant bug will be selected and become the dominant type.

Antibiotics have been used since the late 1940s to fight bacterial infections and disease, enabling millions of lives to be saved. Unfortunately, the extensive overuse and misuse of these drugs throughout the world has allowed resistant strains of

There are some strains of the tuberculosis bacterium (*Mycobacterium tuberculosis*) that are resistant to at least four of the five current antibiotics used against this organism. Because of this resistance, the disease is rapidly becoming a global emergency, claiming over 7,000 deaths per day, worldwide.

deadly bacteria to multiply and to become more prevalent. The animal-food industry has also contributed to this problem. Increased human consumption of antibiotics has occurred indirectly through the practice of feeding them to commercial livestock to increase their overall health and weight gain. The FDA is presently considering a requirement that if a part of an animal's carcass destined for human consumption shows unacceptable limits of antibiotics, the entire carcass must be destroyed. In the past, only the part itself (the liver, for example) had to be eliminated from human consumption.

Antibiotic resistance is particularly important considering the emergence of various antibiotic-resistant strains of bacteria such as *Staphylococcus* in hospitals and other health-care facilities. This emerging issue has stimulated exceptional new efforts among scientists to identify and/or design new drugs. But it takes about eleven years and tens of millions of dollars for a new drug to be developed, approved, and marketed.

One recently developed antibiotic, Zyvox, was approved at the end of 2000 for treatment of various antibiotic-resistant bacteria. The initial targets of the drug include *Streptococcus pneumoniae,* the leading cause of illness and death from infection in the United States, and staphylococcal and enterococcal bacteria, the leading causes of hospital-acquired infections in the United States.

Why is it so difficult to kill a virus?

About the only way to get rid of a viral infection completely is not only to kill the viruses in the tissue and circulation, but also to kill the cells that the virus occupies. None of the antiviral drugs currently available are capable of completely killing all viruses that may be present. As a result, we mainly depend on our own defense mechanisms. However, a few antiviral drugs, acyclovir for example, won't cure us of a herpes simplex virus infection (Type I, the cause of fever blisters or Type II, the cause of genital herpes), but they can significantly help to hold the virus in check. Other agents, like AZT and protease inhibitors, target HIV, the virus responsible for AIDS. Yet others, antiviral agents like amantadine and rimantadine, are effective against the influenza virus Type A strains if taken within two days of onset of the illness. All antivirals do not cure us of the virus, but they do greatly aid our immune system in its work.

Why are there so few antifungal agents?

Antifungal agents are really tough to come by. Most of the drugs that are used to treat fungal infections are very toxic to humans mainly because human cells are very similar to fungal cells with respect to how they work. We can use many of the topical treatments since most fungal infections occur within a limited depth of our skin or mucosal tissues, the outer layer of which normally dies and is shed every day anyway. Drugs such as miconazole are used to treat the fungus that causes athlete's foot.

The problem is quite different, though, if we somehow acquire a fungal infection inside our body. In this case, the infection would be said to be systemic. Although there are antifungal drugs that will work under this condition, these substances are very toxic and require very careful use.

So whether you are taking an antibiotic, an antiviral, or an antifungal agent, keep in mind what these treatments may do to your body. Always discuss any kind of antimicrobial use with your physician. And do not ever take a drug that has been prescribed for someone else.

In Summary

- Wounds, the long-term use of antibiotics, poor nutrition, or a weakened immune system due to situations like disease or because of a particular drug therapy can lead to an opening for a pathogen.
- Antibiotics kill bacteria.
- Antivirals and antifungals kill viruses and fungi, respectively.
- An antimicrobial is anything that kills microorganisms, including bacteria, fungi, and viruses.
- Most antibiotics are made by bacteria and a few are made by fungi.
- Some antibiotics are made from chemicals in the laboratory as designer drugs.
- We can be allergic to an antibiotic.
- Development of resistance to antibiotics among bacteria is rapidly becoming a global problem.

Chapter Six

Our Body—
A Microorganism's Motel 6

From the first moment you emerge from your mother's womb you have acquired the helpful bacteria, fungi, and protozoa necessary for your continuous development. And there are a lot of them: The human body is made up of approximately 10 trillion cells, and a portion of these cells plays host to about ten times as many bacteria. Unlike the exposed surfaces of our body that teem with different microorganisms, the tissues inside of our body do not normally play host to as many living organisms. An exception to this rule is the intestines, which harbor thousands of bacteria that are necessary for us to remain healthy.

Some bacteria, fungi, and protozoa that live within the openings of our body and on our skin provide protection from other, more harmful organisms by occupying limited space and competing for available food. This relationship can be one-sided: We provide nutrients to the organisms and, in return, they do not harm us (this is called commensalism). In other instances, we receive benefits from the germ and the germ gets what it needs from us (this is called mutualism). For example, the *E. coli* bacteria that inhabit our intestines provide us with vitamin K and some of the B-complex vitamins. We in turn provide a place and important nutrients required for these bacteria to survive and grow.

In this chapter we will investigate the nooks and crannies these germs inhabit and explore the ways we can reduce our chances of infection.

The Skin

Our first stop on this journey of the body is the marvelous protective covering known as the skin. The organ with the largest surface area of the human body, the skin is absolutely remarkable: It is pliable but deceptively tough and provides a generally inhospitable place for most of the bad organisms to grow. The outer layer, called the epidermis, is made of continually shedding dead cells filled with a waterproof protein called keratin. New cells make up the second layer and have the job of moving upward, filling with keratin, and dying. The dermis, the third and deepest layer of cells, is loosely attached to the epidermis above it. This tenuous attachment becomes obvious when constant rubbing causes these two layers to separate and fill with fluid—in other words, a blister. The skin as a whole serves as our first line of defense against internal infections.

Is my skin impenetrable?

The skin is not a perfect shield. Bacteria can find their way through this protective cover via sweat glands, oil glands, and hair follicles, all of which have paths from the skin's surface. Even though these routes exist, the area is protected by the secretions from oil and sweat glands and the presence of staphylococci, which combine to generate a slightly acidic (about the level of weak lemon juice) skin surface. Since most bacteria do not grow well on acidic surfaces, this condition helps to protect us from harmful germs.

Is the skin the same everywhere?

The skin's surface properties—those that determine the amount of microorganism growth—vary depending on location. For example, bacteria do not thrive in dry conditions. Therefore, you will find a smaller variety and fewer numbers of bacteria in dry places. However, completely dry conditions do not lead to the absence of bacteria; they may simply cause the bacteria to become dormant. With a little moisture, the bacteria will begin to multiply again.

Skin that is usually moist can be found on the top of the head (scalp), underneath the arms, around the anal region (perianal), and within the ears. A scratch in these areas consequently offers a greater chance for a bacterium to enter the tissues underneath. You know the old adage "Never stick anything in your ear that is smaller than your elbow." Not only can you injure the eardrum, but even a tiny abrasion caused by a fingernail scratch is a large enough site for bacteria to enter. In most cases, an infection in one of these regions is usually localized due to the body's protective defense mechanisms. Nevertheless, one should be aware of the increased vulnerability of moist regions to infections.

Is there a simple way to lower my chance of infection?

Even though the skin of the human body is chock-full of resident microorganisms, we spend our days collecting more. Therefore, it is important to practice good hygiene. One of the best things we can do is to wash the skin, particularly our hands, with plain old soap and water. But washing will not kill every living thing attached to our skin; it only decreases the number of germs on the surface. In a couple of hours the number of germs increases to what it was before we washed.

Most germs that live on our skin are known as residents, or normal skin flora. The majority inhabit the upper layers near the surface, but about 10 to 20 percent can live deep within the epidermal layers. Washing vigorously with standard soaps works well to remove many of these residents and any transient germs that take a temporary ride on the skin's surface. Those that normally reside in the deeper layers are not easily removed by simple washing, but they can usually be killed or inhibited by washing with products that contain antimicrobial ingredients, such as a disinfectant soap. However, you would need to scrub as vigorously and as thoroughly as a surgeon preparing for an operation to kill the germs residing in the deeper layers. So, unless there are special precautions that need to be taken, this kind of intense cleaning isn't really necessary. In fact, the only way truly to sterilize skin is by burning it.

What makes soap antibacterial?

Triclosan is the generic name for an antibacterial agent that is very widely used in household products, and it is now found in some varieties of antibacterial soap, lotion, mouthwash, toothpaste, plastic toys, highchair food trays, socks, underwear, sheets, pillowcases, kitchen sponges, and cutting boards. Similar widely used compounds in bath soaps are triclorcarban and trichlorocarbanilide.

Recent reports from research teams at Tufts University and at St. Jude Children's Research Hospital urge caution regarding the continued widespread use of triclosan. Investigators have identified a bacterium that has built up a resistance to the drug. So avoid overuse of the compounds and be aware that, even though a product may be labeled antibacterial, it does not kill every germ.

Can you ever smell too fresh?

Although everyone likes to smell good, be careful with deodorants. With overuse, you can alter bacteria that hang out underneath your arms and, as a result, increase the risk of infection. Gram-positive bugs, like *Propionobacterium acnes,* release substances that hurt gram-negative bacteria. These substances, as helpful as they are, are also stinky and evaporate into the air, where we can smell them. Therefore, many deodorants are designed to eliminate gram-positive bacteria, such as *Staphylococcus haemolyticus,* thereby reducing the funk. Unfortunately, extremely low numbers of grampositive bacteria make room for gram-negative bacteria to multiply. As a possible consequence of slathering ourselves in deodorant, it may be easier for us to get gram-negative bacterial infections.

While practicing good hygiene is crucial for you and your family's health, do not go overboard. A recent study in Italy quoted in *The New York Times* suggests that creating a superhygienic home environment can actually impair the development of your child's immune system. According to the research, if a child is not exposed to enough dangerous microorganisms, the immune system may become overactive, resulting in the production of antibodies that can result in certain lifelong allergies or asthma.

The composition of most deodorants is very similar, so choose the one that you like best. Since there is little to no research on the substances added to "natural" deodorants, it is not clear how these preparations work to decrease body odor. The chance of infection is slim, so just avoid overuse.

Are pimples caused by bacteria?

These annoying blemishes are usually caused by *Staphylococcus aureus,* a bacterium that enters and establishes an infection at sites beneath the skin in hair follicles. If we have this infection underneath an eyelash, we call it a sty. Normally, pimples are found on the face, but they may occur anywhere a hair is found. If we frequently wash our hands and do not touch our face, we can lower the occurrence of these troublesome inflammations. But sometimes, no matter how hard we try to keep our face clean, stress and normal hormonal cycles can change the makeup of secretions and increase the chances for a pimple to appear.

Every now and then, the bacteria at these sites can grow, spread, and become something known as a boil or abscess. In this case it may be hard for antibiotics to get to the source of the trouble, and we will need to have the blemish opened by a physician. This procedure, along with antibiotics, will usually take care of the infection. Since *Staphylococcus aureus,* the most dangerous of the staphylococci, can cause serious infections within the deeper tissues of the body, keep a good watch on those pimples and if there is concern, see a physician.

Is acne any different from a regular old pimple?

Another more serious condition that is the bane of the teenage years is *Propionobacterium acnes,* which, as you've guessed, causes the disease we know as acne (acne vulgaris). Tiny glands in the skin known as sebaceous glands produce an oil-like substance called sebum. *Propionobacterium acnes* thrive on this substance and as more of it shows up, the bug grows accordingly. The onset of puberty is characterized by an increased production of sex hormones, which also leads to a significant increase in sebum. With the lure of this large food supply, *Propionobacterium acnes* may get involved and the result can be acne—an extensive and damaging skin inflammation. Without treatment, permanent scarring of the face or other parts of the body may occur.

The recommended treatments for acne include vig-

Women should not be pregnant or contemplating pregnancy when beginning Accutane therapy. The manufacturer recommends that sexually active women should use effective contraception during Accutane therapy and for one month after Accutane therapy has stopped. The manufacturer also recommends avoiding all vitamin supplements that contain vitamin A while taking Accutane unless your doctor advises otherwise.

orous cleansing of the skin and application of antibacterial and anti-inflammatory topical ointments. Sometimes antibiotics are also prescribed. A more recent treatment involves a drug similar to vitamin A. This synthetic substance, Accutane, may be prescribed, but with caution, since there may be some pretty rough side effects such as headaches, joint pains, muscle pains, and possible birth defects in infants of pregnant women who are taking the medication.

Are some areas of the skin more susceptible to infection than others?

The skin on the scalp and feet is a little different from the skin on the rest of the body, and both can be plagued by infection just beneath the surface with potential problems from fungi. These fungal infections live on the tissue of the scalp (dandruff), groin (jock itch), feet (athlete's foot), and dead tissue of the nails.

Dandruff, for example, is actually a lay term for scaling, flaky skin on the scalp that is thought to result from an infection caused by the yeast *Pityrosporum,* which grows on the oily secretions of the scalp.

If the fungal infection gets bad, it can sometimes open us up for a bacterial infection too. Since these fungi are thirsty bugs, a person can reduce the chance of infection of the feet or groin by keeping these areas dry. Avoid wearing synthetic underwear and socks; cotton and wool are better because they draw moisture away from the skin's surface. Fungal problems are usually treated with a fungicide (fungus killer). Dandruff needs to be treated with special soaps, many of which are available over-the-counter. If you have dandruff (and lots of us do) do not let anyone else use your hairbrush or comb, and keep these items free of hair and dust by washing them weekly with soap and water.

Nose, Mouth, and Throat

The nose, the mouth, and the areas that make up the throat (called the pharynx) are host to lots of different microorganisms. The mouth is made up of the hard palate, or roof of the mouth, and the soft palate, the tissue that normally closes when we swallow to prevent material from moving into the nasal passages. As you know from having had bubbles in your nose, carbonated soft drinks sometimes get past this barrier. The tissues that lie above and below the soft palate are called the nasopharyngeal (upper, back part of the throat) and oropharyngeal (bottom, back part of the throat) tissues, respectively.

Many of the germs found in these areas can cause problems. For example, *Staphylococcus,* which often lives harmlessly on the skin, can cause abscesses and other serious infections. Another pathogenic organism that is part of our microflora, *Neisseria meningitidis,* can cause an inflammation of the lining that surrounds the brain and spinal cord (the disease called meningitis). Normally a resident in small numbers in the soft palate of an estimated 5 to 30 percent of the U.S. population, *N. meningitidis* can occasionally become active, gain entry into our system, and cause bacterial meningitis. Because many people can carry the disease without becoming symptomatic, outbreaks can appear random. In 1974 and 1975, *N. meningitidis* sickened 250,000 people and killed 11,000 residents of Brazil.

Fortunately, these places—as well as the conjunctiva (eye region) and the gastrointestinal, respiratory, and genitourinary tracts—are lined with a special kind of tissue known as mucous membrane, or mucosa, that is found only where an organ or other tissue has an opening to the outside of the body. The mucus secreted by these tissues makes it difficult for an organism to gain a foothold and therefore protects us.

Behind the soft palate area of the nasopharynx, we can find the germs *Streptococcus pneumoniae, Neisseria meningitidis,* and *Haemophilus influenzae.* The few that congregate in this region are not usually the strains—the encapsulated types—that cause serious illness. Occasionally, dangerous strains of these bacteria can sneak in there and cause serious problems, ranging from pneumonia to an inflammation of the brain.

Teeth

Unlike the soft palate, our teeth are chock-full of bacterial communities: There may be 100 to 300 different species in the little pocket of tissue that surrounds one tooth! Given all of these bugs around the teeth, do not ever share a toothbrush with anyone, no matter how close you are. Whenever we brush our teeth, the germs in the blood from gum tissue and saliva can be transferred to the brush, including things such as hepatitis B and C viruses, oral herpes virus (fever blisters), or HIV. This does not even take into account germs that can be transferred from our hands to the brush. If you have children, teach them not to share a toothbrush. If your toothbrush has been contaminated, simply throw it away and get a new one. Germs do not like dry conditions, so a dry toothbrush harbors fewer germs. After use, always store it in a place where the water can evaporate and replace your brush every few months.

The phrase "getting a little long in the tooth" comes from the fact that as we age, gum tissue often begins to recede, thus making the teeth look a little longer. Some dentists believe bacteria to be the culprits, but others think it is the body's own immune response to bacteria that leads to this tissue loss.

Can the germs from your teeth infect other areas of your body?

The bacteria around our teeth can be of special concern to people with a heart condition known as mitral valve prolapse, especially when they have their teeth

Chewing gum containing xylitol (a kind of sugar alcohol that certain bacteria cannot use) can help control the levels of one of the leading candidates of bacteria associated with tooth decay, *Streptococcus mutans.* According to a study conducted at the University of Minnesota involving 151 patients with high levels of *Streptococcus mutans* around their teeth, the group of patients who chewed gum containing xylitol for five minutes after every meal reduced their levels of bacteria by half, in comparison to the patients who chewed regular gum or sugar-free gum following meals.

cleaned or worked on. Although mouth bacteria are not normally in the bloodstream, little scratches from the dental instruments in the gums or cheeks allow a place for germs to enter. Under normal circumstances, our body easily takes care of the situation, but if a little pocket exists in the mitral valve of the heart where blood pools, bacteria can establish an infection. Be sure to let your dentist know if you have this condition. The presence of an antibiotic in the blood at the time of the procedure will usually protect the individual from the possibility of bacterial infection.

Nose

Although that hair poking out of the openings in our nose can be a little unsightly at times, it serves as an additional layer of protection, trapping germs as well as any duff and dander that might be flying around. A couple of different kinds of bacteria, such as *Staphylococcus epidermidis* and *Staphylococcus aureus,* are often found just inside the flares of the nose. Unless pushed far upward by tissues or fingers, it is unusual for these organisms to travel farther into and establish themselves within the nasal passages and sinuses. If they do cause infection, it is usually grueling and difficult to treat. Consequently, do not use anything—tissues or cotton-tipped swabs included—to probe far inside the nose.

Eyes

Under normal circumstances, it is relatively difficult to contract an eye infection. The first layer of defense is a special protective covering in the white part of the eye known as the conjunctiva, a thin mucous membrane that covers the eye and underneath the eyelids. This membrane, along with blinking, eyelashes (an attractive and efficient physical barrier against bacteria), tears, and mucous secretions, normally keeps the area free from disease. Bacterial infections of the eye are therefore relatively uncommon, mainly because tears contain chemicals and an enzyme that are really tough on germs, especially gram-positive bacteria.

The eye's cleansing system is so efficient that there really is not much more we can do to supplement it, aside from keeping fingers and objects out of there. Each time we touch our eye, we introduce a load of bacteria into the region and increase the risk of scratching the eye. One of the most common eye infections is known as pink eye, which can be caused by different bacteria such as *Staphylococcus aureus* and *Streptococcus pneumoniae,* as well as other bacterial species. The infection is usually treated with eye drops that contain an antibiotic.

Are contact lenses bacteria traps?

The use of contact lenses definitely increases the risk of eye infections. Therefore, carefully follow your ophthalmologist's and optometrist's instructions, as well as those of the manufacturer of your lenses. If you wear a lens for extended periods, various species of *Pseudomonas* can easily contaminate the lenses, causing a serious infection.

Fungi can be a concern with contacts too. *Fusarium* is a fungus that can grow on poorly maintained soft contact lenses. If you see a spot that cannot be removed from the lens, that spot may be a fusarium growth. No matter the type of lens, to keep problems to a minimum, do not prepare your own saline solutions for lens storage. Always wash your hands before handling your lenses and stay within the lenses' recommended wearing time. Always consult with your eye-care personnel prior to doing anything to your lenses, and use good common sense.

What about makeup?

Makeup can also provide a hiding place for germs. Used beauty products are often contaminated with

Pseudomonas, the bacterium responsible for 20 to 30 percent of corneal ulcers. Within a few days of use, eyeliner and mascara can become contaminated, so be careful when applying around the eyes, and never share eye makeup with anyone else.

If an application wand touches the eye, you may scratch the cornea, allowing *Pseudomonas* to enter. An infection of the cornea with this organism takes less than twenty-four hours to cause serious harm to the eye. No matter which bacterium might be the cause, *Staphlococcus, Streptococcus,* or *Pseudomonas,* all infections will normally start to hurt within only a few hours, causing you to do something about it; however, a fungal infection such as those caused by *Fusarium* or *Aspergillus* will not necessarily cause a sharp pain because it acts slowly over an extended period of time—and therefore can cause more damage before it is detected.

To avoid problems, consider buying makeup in small quantities, as the shelf life of most beauty products is usually limited. There are normally preservatives in the makeup, but these substances will deteriorate over time. Following are some guidelines for the shelf life of opened cosmetics:

Mascara, eyeliner, and eye cream: 3 to 6 months
Foundation and face powder: 6 months to 1 year
Cleanser and moisturizer: 1 year
Lipstick and lip liner: 1 to 3 years
Blush and eye shadow: 2 years

Ear

Relative to other parts of the body, the skin inside our ears is moist, and as a result has more bacteria, and therefore, a slightly higher risk of infection. Hair tends to keep germs out of the ear canal, and wax generated within the ear traps infiltrators. Wax also provides a pretty harsh environment that stunts bacterial growth. In the absence of abrasions and the like, daily cleansing of the ears with soap and water is generally sufficient to prevent any bad bugs from taking hold. If you have a wax buildup "problem" in your ear, talk with your physician about the preparations available that can liquefy the wax. These products, if recommended by your doctor, are much safer than scraping around in there every day with a cotton-tipped swab.

Respiratory System

Breathing involves the upper and lower respiratory tracts. The upper tract, an area where bacteria normally reside, refers to the nasal passages, the throat (or pharynx), the trachea, and the very beginning of the tubes (called bronchial tubes) that go into the lungs. The lower tract, which is often bacteria free, includes the lungs and bronchial tissue in addition to the little air-exchange regions inside the lungs known as alveoli.

When we breathe, we immediately offer the inside of our lungs to whatever microorganisms and random dust and particles may be floating by our nose or mouth at the time. And no matter what size nose you may have, each of us takes up to several thousand bacteria into the upper respiratory tract per day. Although these organisms do not usually get past the mucus and those hair-like cilia defenses, there can be an occasional contamination of the lower respiratory tract by bacteria.

We have some neat defenses, though, against such intrusions. Our cough and sneeze reflexes forcefully propel anything that tickles the nose and mouth out of the body. As further defense, any germ that gets as far as the alveoli runs into special cells named macrophages that can kill bacteria. Sometimes, however, germs such as *Streptococcus pneumoniae* enter and grow inside the lower respiratory tract. If a person smokes, or has had a respiratory illness that may have permanently or temporarily damaged the tissues, the organism takes this opportunity to gain a foothold so secure that neither mucus nor cilia can dislodge it. In this circumstance, a germ can multiply significantly, leading to the condition we commonly call pneumonia.

The Gastrointestinal Tract

In the large intestine (colon) all kinds of bacterial reactions take place, and many of them are beneficial to our health. Most of these bacteria are gram-negative and anaerobic, and basically help the body to digest food properly. There are approximately 1 trillion bacteria and more than 300 different species per gram of fecal matter. The usually beneficial bacterium *Escherichia coli,* or *E. coli,* represents only about one-tenth of 1 percent of the organisms in the large intestine.

Can our bodies digest germs?

Regardless of how many germs we swallow, the stomach's acid generally prevents most bacterial growth. Certain bacteria, however, may survive within this harsh soup and get past the stomach into the intestines. For example, one particular stomach survivor, the bacterium *Helicobacter pylori,* is now accepted as the leading cause of stomach ulcers (duodenal and gastric) and is also implicated in stomach cancer. Luckily, this organism can be killed by antibiotics, often making surgery unnecessary. Another bacterium that can cause harm is the acid-resistant strain of *E. coli* (strain O157:H7). Most *E. coli* in our intestines are very helpful and are actually necessary for our good health, but this one member can cause severe diarrhea and kidney damage. We will talk more about this one and related strains when we discuss illnesses associated with food and drinking water.

Other pathogens occur in our intestines, but usually only when something disturbs the amount of germs normally present or changes how all of the occupants interact with one another. The *Clostridium* genus has some pretty mean members, including the dangerous *Clostridium botulinum,* which produces botulism toxin. Even a tiny amount of this toxin in the bloodstream affects how nerves function and can cause paralysis to the extent that a person is unable to breathe. If not properly treated, ingestion of this toxin can cause death. Treatment is usually an injection of antibodies prepared against every known form of the toxin, as well as assistance with breathing until symptoms disappear. While these bacteria do not fare very well in the intestines of adults, the organism thrives in children less than one year of age. Almost all cases of botulism poisoning in the United States are connected to honey being fed to children one year old or younger. Since there isn't any easy way to remove this bacterium from honey or kill it in the honey, all honey is potentially dangerous to infants.

Other opportunists are the bacteria *Clostridium difficele*, which hang around in the intestines but, due to the competition for space and food, do not normally establish themselves. If a relatively long-term antibiotic therapy is used that causes the reduction in numbers of the good bacteria in the intestines, the organism can increase to cause pseudomembranous colitis, a gastrointestinal disease. If you are scheduled to take antibiotics for a long period of time, or to receive high-dose antibiotic therapy for a shorter period of time, discuss this particular issue with your physician.

What germs reside in the areas of the body that eliminate waste?

Under normal circumstances, the kidneys, the bladder, and the tube (ureter) that leads from each kidney to the bladder have no microbial growth. But, as you might expect, the exit end of the urethra, the tube leading from the bladder into the male's penis or particularly into a female's vagina, may contain a few bacterial species.

The vagina has a complicated mix of various bacteria. The number and organization of the bacteria change depending on the woman's age, the menstrual cycle, and with alterations in the acidity of the vagina. One bacterium, *Lactobacillus acidophilus,* ferments a sugar polymer (glycogen) produced by the vaginal tissue into lactic acid. Consequently, both the vagina and cervix are somewhat acidic, and this condition usually inhibits infections.

Men do not have this protection and must depend on the length of the urethra (about twenty centimeters) to provide a distance barrier to the urinary tract. Conversely, the length of the female urethra (about five centimeters) allows for easier access of bacteria to the female urinary tract, which may explain why females are more than ten times more likely than males to experience urinary tract infections.

In Summary

- The enclosed tissues of our body—such as those of the heart, the kidneys, and the liver—that have no surfaces exposed to the external environment are normally sterile, with a complete absence of living microorganisms.
- If a germ happens to gain entry into our tissues, the immune system is activated and will usually remove the intruder.
- The skin is the largest organ (in surface area) of the body and is teeming with germs.
- The skin has different properties on different areas of the body, and, therefore, the kinds of organisms vary depending on the area where the organisms reside.

- Moist areas on the body usually have more microorganisms than drier areas.
- Mucosal tissue is a specialized tissue that makes the protective substance known as mucus that traps bugs.
- Washing with regular soap and water temporarily lowers the number of bacteria present on the skin.
- The commonly used disinfectant triclosan kills bacteria like an antibiotic.
- Overuse of certain antibacterial cleaning agents, such as triclosan, may lead to bacteria that are resistant to these highly effective chemicals.
- Our ability to digest food properly depends in large part upon the bacteria that normally live in our intestines.
- Never feed honey to a child who is one year of age or younger, because of the increased risk of botulism.
- Buy makeup in small quantities because it can easily become contaminated.
- Never share a toothbrush or allow your children to share a toothbrush with another person.
- Clean your nose gently or you run the risk of pushing potentially harmful germs into the deeper nasal passages and causing an infection that can be very difficult to treat.

Chapter Seven

Colds and Flu—You Can Run but You Can't Hide

Unless your job description is "hermit in remote cave," you are probably destined to have close contact with other people on a daily basis. While these interactions are not always fun, at least they aren't always dangerous. But when cold and flu seasons roll around, venturing out can get a little scary, particularly when everyone around us seems to be sneezing and coughing. In this chapter we'll focus on the common cold and the flu, and what you can do (besides becoming a recluse) to avoid them.

What causes the common cold?

The common cold is actually an infection caused by a virus that wreaks havoc on the upper respiratory region. At one time or another, each of us has experienced the stuffy nose that becomes a dripping faucet in between fits of sneezing and coughing, the sore and scratchy throat, and that overall bad feeling. Relative to other respiratory illnesses, cold symptoms build slowly, are generally mild, and may last only a week or two at most, but they can affect our ability to work or to attend school. For those who suffer from asthma or severe allergies, a bad cold can sometimes lead to complications in the lower respiratory tract, including the bronchial tubes and the lungs.

How do we catch colds?

Most colds are caused by one of about 200 identified viruses. Although between 30 and 50 percent of colds are not yet associated with an identified virus, all colds are presumed to be caused by a virus of some sort. Therefore, regardless of the kind of virus that may be involved, the temperature outside has nothing to do with getting sick. In other words, you will not "catch" a cold by going outside naked and making angels in the snow. Although you might be uncomfortable, as long as one of these particular viruses is not present you will

---

From the National Institute of Allergy and Infectious Diseases of the National Institutes of Health: "In the course of a year, individuals in the United States suffer 1 billion colds, according to some estimates. The economic impact of the common cold is enormous. The National Center for Health Statistics (NCHS) estimates that in 1994, 66 million cases of the common cold in the United States required medical attention or resulted in restricted activity. In 1994, colds caused 24 million days of restricted activity and 20 million days lost from school."

not get a cold. The worst the cold weather can do is to inflame the upper respiratory mucosa mildly, making you more susceptible to a viral infection. By the same token, wearing a hat, covering your neck with twenty feet of woolen scarf, and wearing waterproof rubber boots will not prevent a cold if the virus is present.

The flu is a respiratory illness caused by one of three different members (types) of the influenza virus group, Types A, B, and C, with Type C leading to the mildest and least dangerous infection. The viruses that cause influenza, most commonly Type A and sometimes Type B, spread through the air or through person-to-person contact, enter our throat and lung tissues, and begin to multiply. However, in some instances (about 15 percent of the time), colds are due to influenza virus infection (very mild symptoms result). But the normal outcome of this infection can be a lot worse than a cold—a lot worse. In the United States this virus normally begins to appear in the fall of the year, reaches peak activity in December, and usually remains active through the spring of the year. Unlike a common cold, flu symptoms start to appear fairly rapidly, usually within as little as one day after infection, and the symptoms are more serious than those of a cold, including a fever, a cough, and exhaustion. This rapid and more severe response is probably the best way to know whether you've contracted a cold or been really unlucky and gotten the flu. Another clue is that the flu doesn't cause a runny nose.

The flu's attack can be severe: The virus alone can kill a person, but this result is rare if a person is healthy. However, death from complications caused by additional infections by other viruses or, more commonly, by certain bacteria, is of significant concern—even to an otherwise healthy person. The flu viruses can cause extensive damage to the tissue of the bronchial tubes and lungs. Because of this damage, bacteria in particular can much more easily infect the lungs. These additional infections can later lead to a fatal pneumonia. This latter kind of pneumonia (bacterial rather than viral) is usually caused from infection by one or more of these three species of bacteria: *Haemophilus influenzae, Staphylococcus aureus,* or *Streptococcus pneumoniae.* As a protective measure, your physician may prescribe antibiotics to combat a potential bacterial infection. It is for this reason that it is recommended that persons fifty years of age or older receive the flu vaccine but also become immunized against the bacterium *S. pneumoniae.*

In addition to the flu virus, sometimes another virus, called adenovirus, can get in there too. In children, the respiratory syncytial virus can also cause damage to cells and complications due to the changing physiology of the body caused by the ongoing and serious fight against the flu virus. Under these conditions other respiratory-type bugs have a better opportunity to gain an advantage. Consequently, different kinds of respiratory viruses can simultaneously infect a person.

Following are common symptoms of a cold, the flu, and pneumonia. The word *usual* means that this symptom is very likely to occur in every instance. The word *common* means that while the symptom often occurs, it does not happen every time.

Don't Touch That Doorknob!

Symptoms	Cold	Flu	Pneumonia
Runny, stuffy nose	Common	Sometimes	Not usually
Sneezing	Common	Sometimes	Not usually
Sore throat	Common	Sometimes	Not usually
Fever	Unusual	High and sudden	Sometimes high
Headache	Sometimes	Strong	Sometimes
General aches	Some	Usual and sometimes pronounced	Can be quite severe
Cough	Mild, hacking	Can be severe	Frequent and can be severe
Fatigue	Very mild	Extreme, can last several weeks	May happen
Exhaustion	Never happens	Can occur early and be pronounced	May happen
Potential Other Problems	Sinus, ear infections	Bronchitis, pneumonia May be life-threatening	Widespread infection Can threaten life

Why do we catch colds?

According to the National Institute of Allergy and Infectious Diseases, a person's susceptibility to catching a cold is not necessarily related to such things as diet, exercise, or enlarged tonsils or adenoids. However, other research data suggest that psychological stress, allergic disorders that affect the nasal passages or throat, and menstrual cycles may influence a person's susceptibility to catching a cold. It is not known exactly why menstruation makes a woman more susceptible to contracting the common cold, but research indicates that such is the case.

Other factors aside from the ones mentioned above that make people more vulnerable to catching a cold, according to information from the panel of physicians at WebMD (webmd.lycos.com) include the following conditions.

- Exposure to cigarette smoke, toxic fumes, and other air pollutants can damage the cilia in your airways and lungs and can greatly increase your vulnerability to respiratory infections.
- Although colder weather does not cause the common cold, many people do get the majority of their colds in the winter because they are more likely to be indoors, where they are exposed to higher concentrations of rhinoviruses.
- While regular exercise is known to improve health, high-intensity exercise or overexertion may have the opposite effect of temporarily suppressing your immune system, making you more vulnerable to infections.

Cold season does not necessarily correspond with seasonal temperature. The most popular time for the common cold is not during the winter months, a widespread misperception; most colds arrive in fall, spring, and summer (maybe to make room for the flu in the winter). There are so many different cold-causing viruses that most people will not live long enough to acquire immunity to colds. Therefore the younger we are, the more colds we get, because we have immunity to fewer of the cold-causing viruses. Children under the age of twelve have about six or so colds per year, and if the kids are in school, they may have twice as many. Yet people who are more than sixty years old generally have only one cold per year. Adults usually experience between two to four, but women have more than men do, especially if the women are between twenty and thirty years old. It is not actually understood why women at this age have more colds, but one explanation is that they have more frequent and closer contact with young children.

Of the many different viruses that bring on a cold, the usual suspect is one of over 100 different members of a particular kind of rhinovirus (from the Greek word for "nose," *rhinos*) family. Rhinoviruses are estimated to be responsible for about 40 percent of all common colds. When a member of this virus family strikes, the symptoms are usually mild. Other cold-causing viruses such as parainfluenza and respiratory syncytial virus that usually induce mild infections in adults can, however, be severely harmful to kids. Approximately 15 percent of colds are caused by other, potentially more harmful, viruses such as adenovirus, Coxsackie virus, and orthomyxovirus (of which influenza Virus Types A and B are members). The remaining approximately 40 percent of colds are presumably caused by viruses yet to be identified. And, until they are identified, there isn't much we can do about them—except to avoid catching them.

How do I protect myself from catching a cold?

Wash your hands! Wash your hands! Wash your hands! Your kids have to do the same—as often as they can. Do not lick your fingers, rub your eyes, or scratch the inside of your nose before you wash up, because if you have virus on your hands and touch your eyes or mouth or nose, it can pass through the mucous membranes and enter your body. When someone coughs or sneezes, little droplets are expelled into the air (an aerosol), which can contain the active virus. Believe it or not, such particles can remain suspended in the air for hours, remaining active and ready to infect you. Since most of us do not fare too well if we stop breathing, we must depend on a person with a cold not to sneeze openly. If you are around people with colds, and you are not afraid to talk to them, remind them nicely always to cover their mouth whenever they cough or sneeze.

Are doorknobs and other surfaces dangerous to touch during cold seasons?

Cold-causing viruses can remain active for a fairly long time—at least two to three hours—on dry surfaces.

Anytime a person with a cold transfers a virus to a door-knob or something that we may also touch, the active virus can be transferred from the object to our hands, and then to whatever else we touch. Do not use a cloth handkerchief for the sneezes and sniffles. Instead, use tissues and discard them immediately after using. If you work in an office and must use common keyboards or phones, clean the surfaces often with alcohol before you touch them. Taking precautions such as these may seem a little extreme, but if you have asthma or some other respiratory problem that can be made worse by getting a cold, these actions are certainly wise.

Be aware of seemingly innocent transactions we have with people every day. If you are in the supermarket and you notice that the checker has a cold, you are at risk of contracting viruses from the change you receive or the items that are bagged. Keep your hands away from your face and, again, wash them as soon as possible. One defense tip: Carry along some disinfectant wipes (make certain the stuff will kill a virus) for when you cannot find soap or water.

What can we do if we catch a cold?

Antihistamines and other cold remedies may temporarily stop our noses from feeling like a running faucet. However, there is evidence (for rhinoviruses at least) that most of the virus is shed from the nose in those secretions. Usually the first four days or so after getting the cold is when the most viral particles are shed, which makes it more likely for the person who is sick to transmit the virus to another person during this time. So if we stop the dripping nose, we may be less infectious to others.

But at the same time, the overuse of cold remedies can make matters worse. For one, we need to cough and sneeze to expel the virus. If we use a spray to stop our drippy nose, we can dry out the nasal passages so much that the virus can't be eliminated as well, resulting in dry mucosal tissue that can actually make us more vulnerable to a respiratory virus infection. There is also some evidence that taking aspirin may increase the amount of virus that is shed, making it more likely for the aspirin-taking person to infect others. Consequently, there is a balancing act between making yourself feel better versus the potential to make others feel worse. So always discard tissues immediately, cover your mouth when you sneeze, and wash your hands frequently. Here is the latest news from www.drkoop.com on remedies for the common cold:

- *Vitamin C:* There is no evidence that vitamin C has any effect on respiratory viruses.
- *Chicken soup:* The real value of this homemade remedy is its steam. If you are looking for temporary congestion relief, chicken soup is fine, but so is a hot shower.
- *Fluids:* Plenty of fluids are essential for good health, even when you feel great. You should drink six to eight glasses of water or fruit juice every day. Drink extra fluids when you feel a cold coming on.
- *Decongestants:* These over-the-counter treatments really do make you feel better by opening clogged

blood vessels in the upper respiratory tract. Read labels carefully. Be forewarned: Some people experience insomnia or an edgy feeling from some decongestants.

- *Antihistamines:* Yes, they do dry out nasal passages, but they also thicken mucus. So all things considered, they will at least stop your nose from running.
- *Aspirin or acetaminophen:* These are recommended to reduce fever, muscle aches, and joint aches.

Cure for the Cold?

There may be hope on the horizon for treating the common cold, according to results presented at the Second International Symposium on Influenza and Other Respiratory Viruses held in December 1999. A study of a rhinovirus inhibitor drug, AG7088, indicates that it appears to inhibit virus replication. Over one hundred different strains of rhinovirus have been discovered. Another drug under study, pleconaril, has also been shown to interfere with the ability of the cold-causing virus to spread once it has infected human cells. Pharmaceutical companies are involved with extensive human clinical trials (Phase II) to test its effects more thoroughly. If those drugs are approved for human use, the treatment, although not a cure, could measurably reduce the symptoms and shorten the duration of the viral infection.

While aspirin is one of the more effective remedies for fever and other symptoms, a rare but potentially serious condition known as Reye's syndrome can develop when aspirin is taken by young people to help treat any viral infection, including colds and flu. This condition, which has early symptoms of uncontrollable vomiting and nausea, if untreated causes severe brain swelling and inflammation of the liver. Acetaminophen, the active ingredient in Tylenol, was created in response to this syndrome. Therefore, whenever a child younger than fifteen years old gets an infection from a virus of any kind, do not use aspirin in any form—even baby aspirin—to treat a fever or any other symptom. Use caution if you are not sure whether or not it is a virus that is causing the illness. If you have any concerns, talk with the child's physician to get sound advice.

What are my chances of getting the flu?

The Centers for Disease Control states that in an average year, influenza is associated with more than 20,000 deaths nationwide and more than 100,000 hospitalizations. Flu-related complications can occur at any age; however, the elderly and people with chronic health problems are much more likely to develop serious complications after influenza infection than are younger, healthier people.

Why are flu outbreaks seasonal?

Scientists do not understand why flu season begins around the end of October and usually lasts no longer than April. One explanation may be the lower overall temperature of the environment. The influenza viruses generally cause outbreaks of the flu in temperate regions of the world. As the temperature in these regions drops in the fall of the year, it is possible that the flu viruses are able to survive longer outside of a host, such as a pig or bird (the sources of most flu outbreaks), or even a human or two. If the viruses are more active outside a host for a longer time period, there is a greater chance that these viruses can infect a human. As the temperature rises with the approach of spring, the viruses may not last as long outside their animal host. Consequently, the chance of infection by these viruses is decreased.

What is the difference between Types A, B, and C influenza virus?

There are three different major subgroupings, or types, of the influenza virus that we have to worry about. These subgroupings are based on differences in viral protein characteristics. These characteristics are the same for all members within a given type but are different among the three types. As an analogy, humans can be subgrouped into two types, female and male. Characteristics that define humans within a given type are essentially the same, but clearly different between types. While all three types of influenza virus cause the flu, the severity of the illness is determined by which of the three types of virus is contracted. Types A and B are the two major classifications responsible for almost all of the severe cases of the flu. Indeed, a quote from the

CDC states, "Type C infection usually causes either a very mild respiratory illness or no symptoms at all; it does not cause epidemics and does not have the severe public health impact that influenza types A and B do." Consequently, since viral infection by members of the last subgroup, Type C, usually leads to few or no symptoms, this particular subgroup is not the focus of any kind of control measures. A number of different individual strains can exist within each type, particularly Types A and B. So far, Type A is the one that can mutate into a new strain most significantly and rapidly, which has a lot to do with its additional ability to infect species other than humans.

Type B is so far found only in humans, but Type A can be transferred to us from pigs, birds (such as chickens), horses, and even seals. Transmission of the virus from these animals to humans occurs when humans are in close contact with the animals on a day-to-day basis. Animals can cough and spread viruses among themselves and have viruses on them just like we can. If we touch the animal or inhale the virus, we can become infected. Most present-day flu outbreaks begin in regions of the world where farm animals such as pigs and chickens remain in close contact with humans. Once the animal introduces the virus to the human population, further transfer is usually from human to human. Since the Type C subgroup is only rarely responsible for significant illness in humans, identification of this influenza virus is also rare. Anyone infected may show no signs of illness and therefore there is no reason to attempt to isolate the virus for identification purposes. As a consequence, there isn't as much known about the transmission of Type C influenza virus among humans and other animals.

How can I avoid the flu?

Since the influenza virus is so highly infectious, it is very difficult to avoid. The best defense is to get vaccinated. Although the vaccination will not prevent exposure to the flu virus, the chance of infection is greatly reduced—more than 70 percent of people vaccinated do not get the flu. For those who receive the vaccine but become infected anyway, the result is a much milder case of the disease. The success of this vaccination program has led the United States Department of Health and Human Services to recommend that all individuals aged fifty or older (in the past it was sixty-five) receive the flu vaccine every year.

The reason for the recommended vaccination is mostly based on the higher degree of harm experienced by this particular age group during past flu epidemics. The immune systems of older people do not function as

> From the CDC: "Studies have shown the flu vaccine to reduce hospitalization by about 70 percent and death by about 80 percent among the elderly who are not in nursing homes. Among nursing home residents, vaccine can reduce the risk of hospitalization by about 50 percent, the risk of pneumonia by about 60 percent, and the risk of death by 75 percent to 80 percent."

efficiently as those of younger people, making them more susceptible to infection. Once an infection occurs, the weaker immune response allows the infection to be more severe and to last longer, which can potentially lead to bacterial pneumonia, which is caused by *Streptococcus pneumoniae.* Although approximately 90 percent of the severe cases of influenza with complications usually involve this age group, at the same time the vaccine is more than 80 percent effective within this same group.

What exactly is the flu vaccine?

Because the virus can mutate over time, the vaccine itself varies from year to year. Health officials try to predict nine or ten months ahead of time which strains of flu virus are likely to appear in the coming year in order to have vaccine available at least two months before the flu season begins in earnest. The vaccine often includes at least three different strains of virus: Two different strains of Type A and one of Type B that together are predicted to circulate in the approaching flu season.

The vaccine is made by first allowing the virus to multiply in chicken eggs. (This is why people are asked if they are allergic to eggs before receiving the vaccination.) The virus is then highly purified and, after purification, killed. The virus is killed because only a completely inactive form of the virus is presently considered safe for injection in the United States. Dead, completely inactive viruses cannot cause an infection or disease of any kind, but can lead to a protective immune response. Another form, an attenuated influenza virus vaccine, is being prepared and may be used in the future. An attenuated virus is altered in such a way as to keep the virus active (still infectious and able to replicate) but normally incapable of causing disease. Although attenuated viruses do not normally cause disease (except in rare instances like the presently used oral polio vaccine, for example), they will constantly stimulate a person's protective immune response. In extremely rare instances, though, an attenuated virus can revert to a virus that is very similar to the original form prior to attenuation that causes disease. For example, the oral polio vaccine (Sabin vaccine) is responsible for about one case of polio per 2.4 million doses. The disease may occur in the child receiving the vaccine or in an individual who is in close contact with the child. Consequently, the inactivated polio vaccine (Salk vaccine) is recommended for all persons whose immune system is weakened for any reason. Additionally, the inactivated form of the polio vaccine is now recommended (as of 2000) for all children in the United States who are not yet immu-

---

The influenza vaccine should be administered between September and mid-November to ensure the best results. The optimal time for persons at high risk for influenza-related medical complications is usually the period from October to mid-November. It takes about one to two weeks after vaccination for antibodies against influenza to develop and provide protection.

---

nized against the polio virus (see the recommended immunization schedule for children that is provided in Chapter Fourteen). Because of this possibility of reversion of an attenuated virus to a disease-causing form, if an attenuated flu vaccine were approved, some restrictions would likely be applied.

Who in the United States should be vaccinated against the flu?

The CDC makes the following recommendations:
"Influenza vaccine is specifically recommended for people who are at high risk for developing serious complications as a result of Influenza infection. These high-risk groups include:

- All people aged fifty years or older
- People of any age with chronic diseases of the heart, lung, or kidneys, diabetes, immunosuppression, or severe forms of anemia
- Residents of nursing homes and other chronic-care facilities housing patients of any age with chronic medical conditions
- Women who will be more than three months pregnant during the Influenza season
- Children and teenagers who are receiving long-term aspirin therapy and who may therefore be at risk for developing Reye's syndrome after an Influenza virus infection
- Influenza vaccine is also recommended for people who are in close or frequent contact with anyone in the high-risk groups defined above."

Who in Canada should receive the flu vaccination?

The following are general recommendations for persons in Canada who should receive the influenza virus vaccine prepared for that nation:

- Those sixty-five years old and older
- Adults or children over the age of six months suffering with long-term illnesses such as AIDS, anemia, cancer, cystic fibrosis, diabetes, immunological disorders, HIV, heart conditions, kidney disease, lung problems including asthma and emphysema
- Those with a medical condition requiring close supervision of a physician
- Those who have required hospitalization in the past year
- Children six months to eighteen years old who are receiving long-term aspirin (ASA) therapy (Infection of the influenza virus could cause these children to develop Reye's syndrome, a serious disorder that affects the brain and liver.)
- Women who will be in the second or third trimester of pregnancy during the flu season.

If you have any concerns about whether you should have a flu shot, please consult your physician.

How does the flu change every year?

Influenza viruses constantly mutate, so every year can bring a new strain. The mutations lead to changes to the surface characteristics of the virus and therefore make one strain different from another. These differences allow a new form (one not encountered before) of virus, for a time, to evade recognition by our immune system. The "old" antibodies made in response to the old flu strain do not recognize the new flu strain. Even though a protective immune response will eventually occur in the infected person, evasion lasts long enough for this virus to cause an illness to develop.

Can we become immune to the flu?

If we had the flu and survived the disease, or were vaccinated, we would normally be protected against the particular strain of influenza virus involved. But we would not be protected against a different strain, even if the same type of influenza virus infected us. If the flu virus mutates, it takes time for our immune system to respond against the new form, allowing the virus to establish an infection and cause harm before our body can defeat the virus.

The H and N numbers referred to in the following information from the Centers for Disease Control and Prevention are designations for specific viral proteins that appear on the surface of the virus—the "shape" our immune system recognizes. The H stands for hemagglutinin, a flu-virus protein that binds to sugar molecules on our respiratory cells, and the N stands for neuraminidase, which is an enzyme that removes a certain kind of sugar on the surface of our respiratory cells. The type of influenza virus follows the common name for the epidemic (Spanish flu A, for example) and the letters and numbers in parentheses represent the new kinds of these proteins identified.

Here is some pandemic historical information provided by the CDC: "The 1918–19 Spanish flu A (H1N1) caused the highest known Influenza-related mortality: Approximately 500,000 deaths occurred in the United States, 20 million worldwide; The 1957–58 Asian flu A (H2N2) caused 70,000 deaths in the United States; The 1968–69 Hong Kong flu A (H3N2) caused 34,000 deaths in the United States." As you can see, every time a significant mutation occurred, there was an equally significant harmful result, and each time, the virus type was A.

What can I do to avoid the flu?

If you are not able to get a flu vaccination, handwashing is the next best thing you can do. Additionally, try to avoid crowds, especially in enclosed places. But when you must venture out, stay away from coughers if at all possible—coughing is the most common mode of virus transfer other than handled objects (such as money, utensils, cups, and drinking glasses). If you have the flu, stay home and avoid contact with others as much as possible until you are better. Make sure that you keep any children who have the flu away from any elderly persons, even if these people have been vaccinated. The strain of virus that your child has may not necessarily be exactly the same one against which the older people have been immunized. Do not use the same pillow as the person who is ill and wash clothes and bedding more frequently than usual. Whenever possible, use bleach when washing clothing. Also, if you or someone in your home is a high-risk person, you

Make sure the bleach used for disinfectant purposes contains some form of chlorine-based chemical such as sodium hypochlorite. Sodium hypochlorite is the active chemical that disinfects. Therefore, color-safe bleaches should not be used as a disinfectant. Unlike color-safe bleaches, liquid Clorox, for example, contains sodium hypochlorite at a concentration of 5.25 percent. At this concentration of active chemical, one tablespoon of Clorox diluted in one gallon of water is a potent disinfectant.

might consider temporarily using a disinfectant spray, such as diluted chlorine bleach, for toilet handles and doorknobs if there is a case of a cold or flu going around. The bleach kills germs—just leave it on the object for at least five minutes before rinsing. Be sure that any products labeled as disinfectants kill viruses before you purchase them. Have a separate garbage can with a disposable bag for discarded tissues.

Are there additional things I might do to prevent the flu or at least reduce the symptoms?

Yes, if within forty-eight hours of contracting this virus you can be diagnosed by a doctor as having the flu, there are some drugs that may help. Four different compounds are presently licensed for prescription for influenza virus infection symptoms and reduction in disease severity: amantadine, rimantadine, zanamivir, and oseltamivir. When administered as treatment within two days of illness onset in healthy adults, amantadine and rimantadine can reduce the severity and duration of signs and symptoms of influenza virus Type A illness. And zanamivir and oseltamivir can reduce the duration of uncomplicated influenza virus Type A and B illness by approximately one day. Please keep in mind that all currently licensed antiviral agents—including those used to treat influenza virus infection—only inhibit the attachment of the virus to cells or inhibit replication of the virus. None of the currently available substances actually kill the virus.

In Summary

- A cold can make us miserable, but the flu can kill us.
- In 1994, colds caused 24 million days of restricted activity and 20 million days lost from school.
- Most cases of the common cold are caused by one of the over 100 or so different strains of rhinovirus.
- Exposure to cold temperatures does not cause a cold—only viruses do.
- Most colds arrive in fall, spring, and summer—not in winter. Because we are more often indoors in winter, we can more easily transfer cold viruses among ourselves.
- Children have more colds than adults.
- Washing hands is one of the best ways to prevent transfer of cold viruses among us.
- Anyone fifteen years of age or younger should not

take aspirin to treat a fever due to any kind of viral infection, including a cold. A rare but dangerous neurological condition known as Reye's syndrome may result.

• The flu is not a cold. Influenza viruses, usually Type A or B, cause the flu, a significantly more serious condition than a cold.

• The flu is dangerous, and those in high-risk categories that include people fifty years of age or older and people of any age with chronic diseases of the heart, lung, or kidneys, diabetes, immunosuppression, or severe forms of anemia should be vaccinated.

• Vaccination against the flu is recommended for all persons in high-risk groups.

• Along with the flu vaccination, your physician may also recommend that you be vaccinated against *Streptococcus pneumoniae,* the leading cause of severe complications from influenza that leads to bacterial pneumonia.

• There are drugs that can be taken within forty-eight hours of contracting influenza virus—rimantadine, amantadine, zanamivir, and oseltamivir—that may reduce the severity and length of the disease. You may wish to discuss this option with your physician and pharmacist.

Chapter Eight

Water, Water Everywhere—Be Careful What You Drink

In the United States, the chance of serious illness from contaminated water is rare. In this chapter we'll focus on the things we can do to minimize further risk of infection from any harmful bacteria or viruses we may ingest by this route. As there is no place like it, we'll begin in the home, specifically with the water you drink.

Are some people particularly vulnerable to waterborne illness?

If you are generally healthy and your immune system is working properly, you can usually ward off an infection contracted through food or water. The scenario is quite different, however, for certain groups of people.

The people most vulnerable to water- or food-borne illnesses include pregnant women (because of the danger to the fetus), young children, elderly persons, and anyone with a weakened immune system. If anyone in your home falls into these categories, you must be particularly aware and informed. For such a person, a waterborne illness can be very, very dangerous and sometimes lethal.

How safe is the tap water in the average home?

In a world teeming with microorganisms, most of the potentially harmful critters are found in the soil and/or the intestines of animals. Because of surface water's exposure to soil and animals, sophisticated treatment facilities are necessary to ensure that the municipal water supply is safe to drink.

Personnel in city and rural treatment facilities constantly monitor the water supplies, following all sorts of Environmental Protection Agency (EPA) requirements, and they routinely treat the water to prevent contamination. For example, such supplies are tested (often hundreds of times per month) for the presence of bacteria. If bacteria such as *E. coli* or any other fecal coliforms (bacteria common to fecal matter) are within the water supply that leaves the treatment facility, the water is considered to be unsafe. There is a filtration system in

From the Environmental Protection Agency (EPA): "Nationwide, approximately 53 percent of all drinking water comes from ground water sources (wells), with the remaining 47 percent coming from surface water sources (rivers, lakes, and reservoirs). In 1997, 88 percent of the population served by community water systems received drinking water with no reported violations of any health-based standard."

place to remove pathogens (such as the parasite *Giardia lamblia*), and the water is treated to ensure removal of viruses and bacteria. All public water supplies are usually disinfected with a chemical that contains chlorine in one form or another. As a result of these constant efforts and strict policies, the United States has one of the cleanest and safest water supplies in the world.

Even with these precautions, an estimated 900,000 out of the approximately 270 million people in the United States suffer each year from an illness due to contaminated drinking water. Of those stricken, about 900 die. Even in the face of these numbers of illnesses and deaths, you do not have to be a math whiz to calculate that the risk of becoming ill in our nation by this route is quite low. In comparison to the United States, the World Health Organization (WHO) estimates that an average of over 30,000 people die per day as a result of unclean water in developing countries.

What harmful germs reside in water?

Following are disease-causing organisms that can be readily transmitted in water:

- *Campylobacter fetus*
- *Cryptosporidium parvum* (a protozoan)
- *Giardia intestinalis* (a protozoan)
- *Giardia lamblia*
- *Escherichia coli* (pathogenic strains including a particularly dangerous strain, O157:H7)
- Pathogenic strains of *Listeria* (more likely to be found in food)

- *Shigella*
- *Legionella*
- *Salmonella*
- *Staphylococcus*
- Other water-borne organisms include *Yersinia enterolitica* (rare in the United States but more common to Western European waters), *Vibrio cholerae,* hepatitis A virus, and poliovirus.

The majority of the bacterial organisms listed above cause gastrointestinal illnesses either through the organism itself or from the production of toxins by the organism, and some may be severe. For example, *Listeria* can enter the tissue and bloodstream and is capable of infecting the fetus via the mother's blood. In addition to gastrointestinal effects, *Escherichia coli,* strain O157:H7, may also lead to kidney damage and death in the very young or the elderly.

In May 2000, a harmful strain of *E. coli* O157:H7 contaminated the water supply of the rural town of Walkerton, Ontario, Canada. More than 2,000 of the 5,000 residents of the town are thought to have become ill, and approximately 20 people died as a result of drinking the water. At the time of this writing, it has not been determined how the organism entered the water supply, but one theory is that heavy rains could have washed cattle fecal matter into the town's water supply system.

Can all dangerous organisms be killed or safely removed from the water?

Almost all of the organisms that lurk in our water are killed by the filtration systems and the addition of chlorine or chlorine-like agents used in water treatment, with one exception: *Cryptosporidium parvum,* or *C. parvum.* Although thought always to have been in our water systems, this protozoan was identified in 1976 as a human disease–causing agent. A particularly bad outbreak of *C. parvum* occurred in Milwaukee, Wisconsin, in 1993, where approximately 400,000 people became ill and over 100 died. While the vegetative form of this protozoan is susceptible to chemical and other treatments, the cysts of this organism, known as oocysts, are particularly resistant to these same regimens. Unfortunately, along with resistance to standard treatments, *Cryptosporidium* cysts are difficult to identify with presently available testing methods, but better detection methods are currently being developed. Luckily, the incidence of these cysts appearing in municipal water supplies appears to be very low.

For the Web site of the EPA that allows you to see reports on-line of your particular public water supply, state by state and city by city, connect to: http://www.epa.gov/safe water/dwinfo.htm.

If you have questions about your municipal water supply, call the local water department. *All* information about treatment of the water you drink and reports on the water's safety—if it is public water—is open to you. And you might want to take a tour of the facility. If you have children, take them with you. Talk with the people who are responsible for keeping our water safe. I expect that you will be amazed and most likely quite comforted at what is done to make the water safe for you and your family's use.

Is there anything I can do to help protect myself from waterborne germs?

If you are a person with a weakened immune system, there are additional precautions that can be taken to reduce substantially the threat from many of these infectious organisms. Water can be boiled for safety, but the water must remain boiling (at a rolling boil) for at least one full minute (at higher elevations, boil five to ten minutes). This water can be used anywhere you might ingest water, including for brushing your teeth. One potential problem in using boiled water is that any metals or carcinogenic organic substances that might be present already in the water may become concentrated in the process. Low levels of lead, for example, can be concentrated to toxic levels after boiling the water. (Hard to win sometimes, isn't it?) If you are concerned about this possibility, have the water tested for the presence of harmful substances.

How about filtering the water at the tap?

Filtering water from the tap is beneficial, as long as the appropriate system is installed. While some pitcher filtration systems have been proven to reduce the levels of chlorine, sediments, herbicides, pesticides, and other harmful substances, they do not filter out any microorganisms. Some faucet filters have been shown to filter out the harmful microorganisms *Cryptosporidium* and *Giardia*. However, neither pitcher nor faucet filters are intended to purify untreated water, and those individuals requiring water of special microbiological purity should follow the advice of their doctor or local health officials.

Following is information provided by the EPA for home water-supply safety:

"EPA neither endorses nor recommends specific home water treatment units. EPA does register units that make germ-killing claims (contact the National Antimicrobial Information Network at 800-447-6349 for more information). No single unit takes out every kind of drinking water contaminant; you must decide which type best meets your needs.

"For help in picking a unit, contact either of these independent non-profit organizations: NSF International (877-8-NSF-HELP) tests and certifies home water treatment units, and the Water Quality Association (708-505-0160) classifies units according to the contaminants they remove as well as listing units that have earned its approval. Underwriter's Laboratory also certifies some home water treatment units. Water treatment units certified by these organizations will indicate certification on their packaging or labels."

Also, any filter needs to be changed per the manufacturer's instructions because it is difficult to determine when a filter is no longer functional. Even then, filtering may not always assure protection. To filter something like *C. parvum,* the filters must have an *absolute* pore size (not nominal pore size) of less than one micron (that's one-millionth of a meter). Filters designed for cyst removal must remove 99.95 percent of all particles in the 3.0-to-4.0-micron range and should also remove oocysts. If the filters do not have this certification, they are not qualified for the job.

How do I know that my bottled water is pure?

The bottled water industry in the United States is regulated on three levels: federal, state, and trade association. U.S. Food and Drug Administration (FDA) regulations, coupled with state and industry standards, offer consumers a level of comfort that the bottled water they purchase is generally of the highest quality. Federal officials at the Center for Food Safety and Applied Nutrition (CFSAN) with the FDA report that bottled water does not represent any significant health risk.

A recent health report in *The New York Times* and statements from the EPA, however, suggest that drinking bottled water may not necessarily be safer than drinking the water that comes from your tap: Approximately one-quarter of bottled water from major soft-drink manufacturers comes from municipal water sources, and about 20 percent of bottled waters tested had higher bacterial counts than tap water. Additionally, research at Case Western Reserve School of Dentistry and Ohio State University College of Medicine and Public Health revealed that only 5 percent of bottled waters contained the recommended levels of fluoride, which is essential for maintaining good dental health.

The expiration date printed on your bottled water is there for regulatory purposes. Certain states require that bottled water have an expiration date. The U.S. industry standard for the shelf life of bottled water is two years, as long as the bottle is stored in a cool, dark, dry place and not exposed to any solvents or chemicals. The EPA has no regulatory power in monitoring the safety of bottled water. Bottled water is considered to be a food and is therefore regulated by the FDA, but only if the water is sold across state lines. Additionally, each state individually monitors the safety of bottled water produced within that state.

What about distilled water?

Distilled water is prepared by first heating water to the boiling point and then cooling the steam that results. The cooling of the steam returns the gaseous form of water (steam) back to liquid water and the liquid water is then collected in a separate container. Distillation prevents any chemicals that don't become a gas at the boiling point of water from becoming part of the steam. Therefore, distilled water will have much lower amounts of things like calcium, iron, and solid particles (fewer total dissolved solids, or TDS) relative to regular water. Some manufacturers also pass the distilled water though a post-distillation charcoal filtration process. The charcoal helps to remove any organic materials that may have been in the steam. But, just like any other kind of bottled water, remember that the purity and safety of distilled water depends upon the manufacturer.

Are there special concerns about well water?

Those who depend on private well water or any other nontreated source for their home's water have an increased risk for illness. These individuals should frequently have their water tested for the presence of potentially disease-causing organisms. If areas nearby have a number of animals present, either domestic or wild, this examination is particularly important. Sometimes there may be cattle feedlots, animal rearing facilities, etc., that may not be on your property but near your property. If runoff from these areas (surface water) can reach a stream or underground water, however

---

For owners of private drinking water wells, the EPA provides the following information:

"EPA's Safe Drinking Water Hotline provides access to publications and technical assistance over the phone at 800-426-4791. Among EPA's publications that may help you is the detailed *Manual of Individual and Non-Public Water Supply Systems* (EPA 570/9-91-004). Hotline staff may be able to direct you to sources of state and local assistance." For more information, please see EPA's well-water Web site at: www.epa.gov/safewater/pwells1.htm.

---

unlikely, fecal contamination may occur. This runoff may ultimately lead to the presence of potentially harmful organisms within the home's water supply.

What precautions should I take when I have a well dug?

Any well must be properly drilled, constructed, and maintained in order to minimize the contact of surface water with underground water. Anytime a well is dug or a pump is placed into a free-flowing stream to provide water for a home, the water should be thoroughly tested for the presence of disease-causing organisms and harmful chemicals. Test for the presence of such things as nitrates, nitrites, or pesticides (especially in farming areas), and, possibly, radioactive materials, in addition to lead, mercury, and/or carcinogenic substances in the water. There are a number of agencies that can supply information and personnel within them who can perform proper testing of the water. Your county's health department or county extension agency (of the USDA) are particularly important initial sources of information and help, so do not hesitate to use their expertise.

What are the repercussions of natural disasters, such as flooding, on the water supply?

One last note on water supplies: Flooding or other disasters can spread contamination of all kinds throughout a very large area, and these contaminants can enter streams, rivers, reservoirs, and perhaps underground water over time. Aside from the chemicals (agricultural and otherwise) that may be present in floodwater, very harmful organisms such as *Vibrio cholerae* can be present in concentrations sufficient to cause severe illness. Hepatitis virus Type A and other viruses, as well as other dangerous bacterial organisms, are more prevalent because septic systems and sewage drainage systems will overflow.

So stay away from floodwater if possible. If you must be in it, protect yourself as best you can with rubber boots, gloves, and the like in order to prevent ingestion or entrance of organisms through a wound in the skin. Clean everything that comes in contact with the water with diluted bleach (one part in ten is the recommendation from FEMA) or its equivalent.

If there is a flood or other emergency, how do I get safe water?

If there is a flood or any disaster that upsets the water supply in your area, take particular precautions drinking or bathing in that water. Local health authorities will monitor the water supply and issue precautionary steps to the public, but don't wait for an announcement when such conditions exist.

One source of safe water will likely be the American Red Cross and various local health agencies. But, in a pinch, following are instructions from the Federal Emergency Management Agency (FEMA):

After a disaster, it is possible that water supplies will be temporarily cut off or become contaminated. Because you must have water to survive, it is important to know how to locate and purify drinking water to make it safe.

In the home:

- Melt ice cubes.
- Hot-water tank: Turn off the power that heats it, and let the tank cool. Then place a container underneath and open the drain valve at the bottom of the tank. Do not turn the tank on again until water services are restored.
- Toilet tank: The water in the tank (not the bowl) is safe to drink unless chemical treatments have been added.
- Water pipes: Release air pressure in the plumbing system by turning on the highest faucet in the house. Then drain the water from the lowest faucet.

Outside the home:

- Rain water, spring water, and water from streams, river, lakes, and coiled garden hoses can be used after it is purified.

In Summary

- The public drinking-water supply in the United States is one of the safest sources of drinking water in the world.
- Pregnant women (and the fetus), the elderly, the very young, and anyone with a weakened immune system are more vulnerable to harm from pathogen-contaminated water.
- Wells should be frequently monitored for bacterial and viral contamination.

- Boil water for at least one full minute (at high elevations, boil water at least five to ten minutes) to kill harmful bacteria and many viruses.
- Living organisms are not the only concerns with drinking water—chemicals can also be dangerous (copper and lead are two important ones).
- Heavy rains can lead to runoff that can lead to contamination of local water supplies. In these cases, the water district may add additional purifiers to the drinking water.
- If an area is flooded, never swim or play in this water.

Chapter Nine

If You Can't Stand the Germs, Stay Out of the Kitchen

The facts are in, and the news is not good: If you want to find truly terrible germs, you need only look in the kitchen. A number of studies have proven that, without exception, the kitchen wins hands-down as the most germ-ridden room in the house. A University of Arizona study found 300 germs per square centimeter of kitchen countertop. On the surface, this information does not seem to make much sense—the kitchen probably gets more daily cleaning than any other room in the house. However, there are dangers lurking in places that might surprise you: inside the refrigerator, in the sink, in the sponges we use to clean—you name a place, and germs can be found there. Basically, we are dealing with a bunch of freeloaders and squatters that love your kitchen; to them it is home sweet home.

Where do all of these germs come from?

Germs can be hiding on the fresh fruit and vegetables, on or in meat and even in the fresh eggs you buy. Pretty much anything that is not cooked—and sometimes things that are—has the potential to spell trouble.

However it is only when these germs infect us that we can be in danger. Thank goodness our natural defenses are so strong that infection isn't that easy! If we eat food that contains certain bugs on or in it, we can catch what is known as a food-borne illness, or food poisoning. The consequences can be awfully uncomfortable at best, and at worst they can kill us.

The Centers for Disease Control and Prevention (CDC) estimates that food-borne diseases cause approximately 76 million illnesses, 325,000 hospitalizations, and 5,000 deaths in the United States each year. Out of all of the microorganisms that can cause disease, an overwhelming percentage of food-borne illness is caused by some bad bacterium.

Because food rather than water usually causes such illnesses, you need to be diligent about food safety. You need to look at how food is handled, prepared, and stored in the kitchen and find out about the potentially dangerous critters that may be throwing parties inside the refrigerator or building condominiums inside that sponge or dishrag.

What is a food-borne illness and how do we get one?

The overwhelming majority of such illnesses come from introducing a microorganism into our intestinal tract by eating something that is contaminated. We can also ingest the bug by touching our fingers to our mouth after we have actually touched something that is contaminated, including a surface of a container, a piece of fruit, a vegetable, or even on a package that we bring home from the store. So the first thing we can do to reduce the risk of exposure to any hitchhiking critters is to wash our hands, frequently and well, whenever we are exposed to food or food packaging. You cannot simply show the water and soap to your hands; you need to wash them for at least twenty seconds to get full benefit of your efforts.

Which bugs should we be worried about?

In almost all instances of food poisoning, the culprits are bacteria rather than viruses. The most common kinds of microorganisms associated with food-borne illnesses include:

- *Clostridium botulinum*
- *Campylobacter jejuni*
- *Clostridium perfringens*
- *Cryptosporidium parvum*
- *Escherichia coli*, including the harmful strain O157:H7, as well as others
- *Listeria* and *Salmonella*
- *Staphylococcus*
- *Yersinia enterolitica*, which is rare in the United States but more common in western Europe
- The Norwalk virus

Of these organisms, we are most likely to run into one of the harmful strains of *Campylobacter, Salmonella, Escherichia coli,* or *Listeria*. Some of these bacteria cause problems on their own, while others can release substances such as toxins that can harm us even if the bacterium that released them is no longer present.

Is everybody at risk?

Well, to some extent, yes. Any healthy person who gets enough of these harmful organisms inside them can experience gastrointestinal upset, fever, nausea, vomiting, and diarrhea. A person may have one or all of these symptoms, depending on the severity of the infection, and the symptoms may be mild to severe. The amount necessary to make a person sick varies significantly among the germs. Also, the combination of the germs with the health and the age of the person involved can greatly influence whether a person becomes ill. The length of time and the severity of the illness can also vary. People in high-risk groups should be particularly wary of getting food poisoning because the results can be fatal.

If I get "food poisoning," what are some of the symptoms and how can I treat it?

Symptoms of the most common food-borne illnesses are nausea, possibly vomiting, abdominal pain, mild to severe diarrhea, and sometimes a fever. In general, symptoms appear anywhere from twelve hours to two weeks after infection. The length of time depends on a variety of factors, including the amount of the germ encountered, your state of health at the time, your age, and the specific germ involved. If the bug is *E. coli* O157:H7, there may not be any symptoms at all, even though you could have been infected for a while. A bug like *Listeria* occasionally causes gastrointestinal upset or diarrhea but more often causes muscle ache (stiff neck, for example) and fever. And for this organism, it may take as long as two months for the symptoms to show up.

111

In most cases, if you are healthy, the infection will clear after several days without medical treatment. Your immune system will kick in and take care of the problem, but contact a physician anyway, no matter how insignificant you may feel your particular illness to be. Now and then these bugs can fool us with symptoms that are not severe. Germs like *Listeria* or *Salmonella,* for example, can sometimes move from the intestines to infect other parts of the body. So caution is the best policy. If blood appears in diarrhea, immediately contact a physician, especially if the ill person is elderly, a child or an infant, or within a vulnerable group.

Dehydration, a loss of fluid from severe diarrhea due to food poisoning, can lead to kidney failure as well as other damage. The medical community recommends that a person drink fluids until all of the symptoms have disappeared. If you are unsure if you are dehydrated, ask yourself the following questions: Are the insides of my eyelids moist? Does my mouth feel dry? Can I spit? If the answers are no, yes, and no, speak with your physician right away.

What can I do when I contract a food-borne illness?

Contact your physician whenever you suspect that you may have contracted a food-borne illness. Your physician may wish to isolate fecal samples in order to identify the bug involved in case antibiotic or other treatment may be necessary. The CDC Web site in Health Topics A–Z, Health Topic: Foodborne Illnesses at www.cdc.gov details the treatments for the most common food-borne illness. It is excerpted below:

- *Campylobacter:* Virtually all persons infected with *Campylobacter* will recover without any specific treatment. Patients should drink plenty of fluids as long as the diarrhea lasts. In more severe cases, antibiotics such as erythromycin or a fluoroquinolone can be used, and can shorten the duration of symptoms if they are given early in the illness. Your doctor will make the decision about whether antibiotics are necessary.
- *Cryptosporidium:* There is as yet no effective treatment for this illness. Most people with a healthy immune system will recover on their own. Antidiarrheal medicine may help slow down diarrhea, but consult with your health-care provider before taking it.
- *E. coli* O157:H7: Most persons recover without antibiotics or other specific treatment in five to ten days. There is no evidence that antibiotics improve the course of disease, and it is thought that treatment with some antibiotics may precipitate kidney complications. Antidiarrheal agents, such as loperamide (Imodium A-D), should also be avoided.
- *Salmonella: Salmonella* infections usually resolve in five to seven days and often do not require treatment unless the patient becomes severely dehydrated or the infection spreads from the intestines. Persons with severe diarrhea may require rehydration, often with intravenous fluids. Antibiotics are not usually necessary unless the infection spreads from the intestines, then it can be treated with ampicillin, gentamicin, trimethoprim/sulfamethoxazole, or

ciprofloxacin. Unfortunately, some *Salmonella* bacteria have become resistant to antibiotics, largely as a result of the use of antibiotics to promote the growth of feed animals, such as cattle.

- *Listeria:* When infection occurs during pregnancy, antibiotics given promptly to the pregnant woman can often prevent infection of the fetus or newborn. Babies with listeriosis often receive the same antibiotics as adults, although a combination of antibiotics is often used until physicians are certain of the diagnosis. Even with prompt treatment, tragically, some infections result in death.

How do we keep germs to a minimum in the kitchen?

Every time we clean the kitchen counter with a sponge, we collect more and more organisms inside of it. Every time you do something as simple as placing fresh vegetables on the counter or dropping and breaking an egg in the sink, there is a chance for bacterial contamination of these surfaces and, consequently, you as well. Cross-contamination is responsible for 36 percent of the approximately 76 million food-borne illnesses that occur annually in the United States.

With potential trouble lurking on every surface, what do you do? Some simple but effective measures: Clean surfaces you touch constantly, such as the sink faucet and the cabinet handles. Although there are a number of different cleaning products available that reduce bacteria, a diluted solution of bleach (one full teaspoon, about five milliliters, of concentrated bleach to one quart, about 0.95 liters, of water) is a simple and effective way to kill germs. As long as the bacterium isn't a spore, bleach will kill it. And since an average-size sponge or dishcloth can harbor up to 7.2 billion germs, you should soak them in bleach fairly often—at least once a week in general, and especially after cleaning a surface that has been touched by any kind of raw meat or vegetables. This same solution can be used to clean all of the flat surfaces in the kitchen, including the sink and the stovetop. If you want to store the sponges or dishrags after soaking them in bleach, rinse them with water and let them dry.

A good method for killing critters inside sponges and rags is to, as kids would say, "Nuke 'em!" While a sponge or rag is damp—not soaking wet—place one item at a time in a microwave oven and zap it with full power for at least three to four minutes. If the sponge or rag is dry, zap for at least one full minute. This unkind treatment will normally kill most bacteria and viruses. One caution: Do not put any food in the microwave with the sponge or rag—you do not want anything flying around in there to land on the food. You can also put your sponge in the dishwasher and run it. The hot water will kill most germs.

The garbage disposal is another highly concentrated area for germs. (Just think of what goes down there!) Bleach, which is quite potent, can be used here as well. Add a good volume of the bleach solution or antibacterial cleanser to it—do not be chintzy—and let it sit for at least five minutes. Then run the disposal with plenty of water. One thing to remember is that bugs can congregate inside the disposal, and when it is turned on, little droplets can fly out and contaminate surfaces. So clean the disposal *first,* before you clean the sink and nearby counter. Be careful that these droplets do not get into your eyes—no peering down into that dark hole while the disposal is running.

If your countertops will be damaged by bleach, thoroughly and frequently scrub them with a good dish-washing detergent. Further, *never* place raw meat on a countertop made of wood. You may wish to consider cleaning agents that contain phenolic compounds (like cresol) that can inhibit the growth of bacteria. However, carefully examine the manufacturer's recommendations for use of such substances on wood. Residues may accumulate that can irritate the skin and that may also, in time, discolor the wood.

A final note: When you have a particularly germy mess, consider using paper towels or disposable rags to clean it. By throwing out the towel or rag when you are done, you will eliminate the chance for cross-contamination.

How about cutting boards—are they safe?

Yes, if you take care to clean them properly. Plastic and wood each have advantages and disadvantages: One of the first studies determined that wood is easiest to keep clean, but a more recent study found that there was not much difference between wood and plastic with respect to potential for contamination. If either type of board is heavily scratched or gouged, consider replacing it. Bacteria settle into the nooks and crannies and may become dormant, only to awaken inside you later. No matter the makeup of the board, do not let food juices dry before cleaning it. To kill germs below the surface, place the wooden board—best if wet—in the microwave for at least ten minutes (800 watts). Those bad bugs will be boiled alive. As for a plastic cutting board, whether dry or not, no amount of rubbing with detergent will remove the bacteria from the little crevices. But plastic can be treated with a dilute bleach solution, whereas wood reacts with the bleach and destroys its ability to kill anything. Plastic boards can also be placed in the dishwasher and, if the temperature is right, the washer's heat will kill the bacteria. So as long as they are cleaned properly, either kind of board will be safe to use.

What about utensils?

The same precautions should be taken with plastic and wooden utensils as with plastic and wooden cutting boards. Those rubber spatulas or spreaders should be cleaned in the dishwasher or washed thoroughly with soap and hot water. Never use the same utensil for serving that you used to prepare the food. Stainless steel utensils are easier to keep clean because germs cannot grab on to this surface as easily. But if any food remains, bugs will grow and multiply. So again, do not allow utensils to hang around too long before they are cleaned.

How do we clean dishes effectively?

If you wash by hand, make sure to do the dishes within two hours of eating from them and use hot water. Try not to simply rinse the dishes and leave them wet in the sink for too long. Having both water and food rem-

117

nants around at the same time provides good conditions for bacterial growth. Use the same sort of common-sense approach with your dishwasher as well. Do not let the dishes stand around too long and try to keep them relatively dry until washed. Make sure that the water temperature of your dishwasher is at least 140 degrees Fahrenheit. Most dishwashers should have a thermostat that heats the water to the proper cleaning temperature. If you are not sure about the water temperature, and especially if there is an at-risk-group member in your home, have a dishwasher service person check to see if the water is getting hot enough to kill germs.

How should we clean the floor?

Simply put, keep dust and dirt to a minimum: Germs like to travel along with these particles. Wash the floor first with soap and water and let dry before cleaning with the bleach solution. Be sure to read carefully any instructions listed by the manufacturer of the bleach. And be sure to test a small section of the floor to see if there is any discoloring effect as a result of applying this solution—you certainly do not want to ruin your floor. If you have unusual flooring, you may wish to check for commercial floor-cleaning products that will hold the bacteria to a minimum without damaging its surface.

How can I keep the kitchen from getting contaminated by more germs?

The bacteria that cause food poisoning are most often associated with dairy products, eggs, meat, and poultry, as well as cold cuts, fish, and shellfish. These products may be contaminated during slaughter and processing, leading to disease if they are undercooked, mishandled, or temperature abused. So if any of these bugs happen to be present, their numbers can easily grow to dangerous levels in a few hours at the right temperature, making these foods a high risk.

Most bacteria grow between about 41 degrees Fahrenheit (5 degrees Celsius) to about 140 degrees Fahrenheit (60 degrees Celsius), but the majority of pathogens multiply best at body temperature. Do not store any food, and particularly those mentioned above, at or between these temperatures. Even if the items were at room temperature when you bought them, some prepackaged items or containers usually do require refrigeration after opening. The important things are to prepare, store, and cook your food safely and continue to keep the kitchen clean as you go along.

When it comes to food safety, consumers have higher expectations of other food handlers than they do of themselves. According to a survey conducted by Audits International across the country in late 1997, when people prepared meals in their own kitchens, they failed to follow food safety and sanitation practices over 99 percent of the time. These practices included hand-washing, preparing and storing ingredients at proper temperatures, and avoiding cross-contamination.

Is refrigeration really all that important?

You bet it is. Food is not sterile, so with bacteria it is a numbers game before and after the food is cooked. For example, if just one food-poisoning bacterium latched on to a hot dog, it would take only seven hours at the right temperature to increase to more than 2 million. Yikes! That is why you should be sure that the temperature of the refrigerator is below 40 degrees Fahrenheit (35 to 40 degrees is recommended). While this temperature will not kill the bugs, it will slow their growth in the fridge.

A 1997 survey by Audits International encompassing eighty-one cities in the United States of homes where residents knew they were being evaluated found that approximately 20 percent of homeowners maintained their refrigerator temperature above 45 degrees Fahrenheit, and more than 40 percent stored food between 42 and 45 degrees Fahrenheit—both risky situations. Most fridges have temperature gauges, but if yours does not, get a thermometer and check it. If you do not have a thermometer, there is another way to insure that your fridge is cold enough. Adjust the knob until lettuce freezes, then turn the knob to a slightly warmer setting. While the lettuce-freeze test is not ideal, it is better than just guessing. Also keep in mind that you will probably need to adjust the temperature regulator knob as winter turns to summer.

Any frozen food should be kept at 0 degrees Fahrenheit (−18 degrees Celsius) or below. Again, if you do not know the temperature of the freezer compartment, try to find out. Frozen goods need to stay frozen.

While any bacteria that harm you are not killed at this temperature, they do not multiply as often, either. When the freezer door is opened and closed frequently, warm air gets in the freezer, increasing the temperature. And since most freezer compartments in refrigerators are frost-free for convenience, the freezer compartment must warm up now and then to melt the frost. The usual system employs heating coils that cycle on about every six hours to melt the frost. As the temperature inside the freezer approaches 32 degrees Fahrenheit, the heating coils shut off. All of the recommended storage times for frozen food, however, are based upon a constant 0 degrees Fahrenheit. Because of such situations, it is not as safe to store foods in frost-free freezers for long periods of time. Since different kinds of food require different freezing conditions, it is impossible to come up with a tried-and-true food-storage time limit for your particular frost-free freezer. Therefore, the best thing to do is to keep frozen foods no longer than the maximum time recommended for the item if stored at 0 degrees Fahrenheit.

A deep freeze usually does not have this frost-free feature, nor does it experience frequent entry. So the food will remain at a constant, safe 0 degrees Fahrenheit. Take a look at the following recommended refrigerator and freezer storage times for all kinds of food items from the Partnership for Food Safety Education's Web site (www.fightbac.org).

Food	Refrigerator (40°F)	Freezer (0°F)
Eggs		
Fresh, in shell	3 weeks	Don't freeze
Raw yolks, white	2–4 days	1 year
Hard-cooked	1 week	Doesn't freeze well
Liquid pasteurized eggs or egg substitutes		
opened	3 days	Don't freeze
unopened	10 days	1 year
Mayonnaise— commercial (Refrigerate after opening)	2 months	Don't freeze
TV dinners, frozen casseroles	Keep frozen until ready to serve	3–4 months
Store-prepared (or homemade) egg, chicken, tuna, ham, macaroni salads	3–5 days	None of these products freeze well
Pre-stuffed pork & lamb chops, chicken breasts stuffed with dressing	1 day	Does not freeze well
Store-cooked convenience meals	1–2 days	Does not freeze well
Commercial-brand vacuum-packed dinners with USDA seal	2 weeks, unopened	Does not freeze well

If You Can't Stand the Germs, Stay Out of the Kitchen

Food	Refrigerator (40°F)	Freezer (0°F)
Soups & Stews Vegetable or meat-added	3–4 days	2–3 months
Hamburger & stew meats	1–2 days	3–4 months
Ground turkey, veal, pork, lamb & mixtures of them	1–2 days	3–4 months
Hot dogs		
Opened package	1 week	1–2 months
Unopened package	2 weeks	1–2 months
Lunch meats		
Opened	3–5 days	1–2 months
Unopened	2 weeks	1–2 months
Bacon & Sausage		
Bacon	7 days	1 month
Sausage, raw from pork, beef, turkey	1–2 days	1–2 months
Smoked breakfast links, patties	7 days	1–2 months
Hard sausage, pepperoni, jerky sticks	2–3 weeks	1–2 months
Ham, Corned Beef		
Corned beef in pouch With pickling juices	5–7 days	Drained, wrapped, 1 month

Don't Touch That Doorknob!

Food	Refrigerator (40°F)	Freezer (0°F)
Ham, canned— label says keep refrigerated	6–9 months	Don't freeze
Ham, fully cooked— whole	7 days	1–2 months
Ham, fully cooked— half	3–5 days	1–2 months
Ham, fully cooked— slices	3–4 days	1–2 months
Fresh Meat		
Steaks, beef	3–5 days	6–12 months
Chops, pork	3–5 days	4–6 months
Chops, lamb	3–5 days	6–9 months
Roasts, beef	3–5 days	6–12 months
Roasts, lamb	3–5 days	6–9 months
Roasts, pork & veal	3–5 days	4–6 months
Variety meats— tongue, brain, kidneys, liver, heart, chitterlings	1–2 days	3–4 months
Meat Leftovers		
Cooked meat and meat dishes	3–4 days	2–3 months
Gravy and meat broth	1–2 days	2–3 months
Fresh Poultry		
Chicken or turkey— whole	1–2 days	1 year
Chicken or turkey pieces	1–2 days	9 months
Giblets	1–2 days	3–4 months

Food	Refrigerator (40°F)	Freezer (0°F)
Cooked Poultry—		
Leftover		
Fried chicken	3–4 days	4 months
Cooked poultry		
dishes	3–4 days	4–6 months
Pieces, plain	3–4 days	4 months
Pieces covered with	1–2 days	6 months
broth, gravy		
Chicken nuggets,		
patties	1–2 days	1–3 months

Do cold temperatures slow the growth of all bacteria?

Unfortunately, no, not all. The bacterium *Listeria monocytogenes,* one of the most dangerous, is notoriously resistant to refrigeration. This bacterium will actually grow, although slowly, at proper refrigeration temperature. Potential sources of *Listeria* include such foods as non-pasteurized milk, cheeses (particularly those that are soft-ripened), ice cream, raw vegetables, raw meats (essentially all types), and smoked and raw fish. Contamination is possible even if the food is commercially packaged. This bug can cause severe infections among those with compromised immune systems.

Among vulnerable populations, particularly at risk is the fetus within a pregnant woman. An otherwise healthy pregnant woman can be infected with *Listeria* and have no symptoms at all. Estimates suggest that a pregnant woman is about twenty times more likely than a non-pregnant woman to become infected by this organism, even though the woman may be otherwise completely healthy. She may also show no signs of illness whatsoever, but any bugs inside her bloodstream can cross the placenta and infect the child. Some doctors recommend that all cold cuts, regardless of whether they are processed, should be avoided during pregnancy.

Because of the danger of *Listeria* infection in at-risk groups, the U.S. Department of Agriculture (USDA) in May of 1999 recommended that extra precautions be taken in food preparation: All ready-to-eat food such as luncheon meats, hot dogs, deli meats, cold cuts, various dry and fermented sausages, along with other meats and poultry products, should each be reheated until steaming hot before eating.

So if you really want to eat it, you had better heat it. Otherwise, the USDA recommends that at-risk groups not eat these foods at all. Other refrigerated foods that vulnerable groups are recommended to avoid: various soft cheeses that include Camembert, Brie, blue-veined cheese varieties, and types of soft Mexican-style cheese (such as queso fresco and queijo fresco, for example).

I know, you may really love one or all of these things, but eating any one of these foods can be taking a dangerous gamble. Fortunately, not all cheeses are dangerous. The USDA says that at-risk groups can safely eat hard cheeses, processed cheese, cream cheese, cottage cheeses, and yogurt.

Are there dangers associated with thawing frozen foods?

Thawing food as quickly as possible is a good idea, so plan ahead. Move frozen food from the freezer to the refrigerator. Leave food in a sealed container. Let it hang out there for several hours before you move it to the countertop or microwave for thawing. If the item is large or dense and won't fit into a microwave oven, place the item in a warm-water bath and change the water every ten to fifteen minutes. Here is a hard and fast rule: do not thaw and then refreeze uncooked meat. Here is why. Freezing makes ice form inside the cells and, since water expands upon freezing, the cells rupture, nutrients leak out, and bugs love the nutrients. You get the picture—bacteria-o-rama.

How do you refrigerate cooked foods properly?

Any cooked food that will be immediately refrigerated or frozen should be stored while hot in small, shallow portions to allow the contents to cool rapidly. Any deep-dish food should be transferred to shallow containers before refrigeration or freezing. Otherwise, the food could remain warm in the center of the dish for over the two-hour time limit, and microorganisms could grow there before the temperature dropped to a safe storage or freezer temperature.

What about cooking requirements?

When preparing any kind of meat, be especially aware of the potential health problems. *Campylobacter, Listeria, E. coli,* and *Salmonella* are bacteria that can be associated with meat products—and I mean closely associated. For example, it is estimated that as many as 500 bacteria may be present in only one drop of poultry juice, and that 60 percent or more of raw poultry on sale to consumers contains some disease-causing bacteria.

The only way to be sure that meat gets hot enough to kill germs is to use a thermometer. When cooking an entire bird, make sure the internal temperature reaches at least 180 degrees Fahrenheit (82.2 degrees Celsius). A steak should reach at least 145 degrees Fahrenheit (62.8 degrees Celsius) on the inside.

Ground meat—e.g., hamburger—can be a particular problem. When meat is ground, any *E. coli* O157:H7 or other bacteria that may be present on the outside of the meat will become distributed throughout the hamburger. Consequently, ground beef should be cooked to well done, with a minimum internal temperature of 160 degrees Fahrenheit. So if you like your hamburgers walking-off-the-plate rare, you are increasing your chances for infection.

The same concerns surround regular pork and chicken breasts or fillets. All of these foods should be cooked to an internal temperature of at least 160 degrees Fahrenheit (71.1 degrees Celsius). Use a meat thermometer or those little temperature sticks that change color when the correct temperature is reached. If you do not use any kind of mechanical temperature test, make sure that the juices run clear—not pink, not sort of clear, but *clear*.

If you have any additional questions about safe cooking techniques, call the USDA Meat and Poultry Hotline (800-535-4555).

What is it about E. coli *that makes it so dangerous?*

Most members of the *E. coli* family are essentially harmless. But there are several culprits among them that are really bad germs. Each of the different harmful strains produces its own brand of toxin. Some of these toxins are worse than others are, but all can be harmful to some extent. Each is a protein that generally produces mild to severe diarrhea, but some of them can cause severe damage to intestinal cells and blood vessels.

The strain O157:H7 is particularly dangerous—and this is the one you have read or heard about most frequently. Each year in the United States, several deaths result from the approximately 100,000 illnesses thought to be caused by the O157:H7 strain. Many thousands of pounds of meat have been recalled in attempts to protect the consumer. Recent studies have estimated that a whopping 50 percent of our nation's beef supply is contaminated with the O157:H7 strain, an amount ten-fold greater than previously estimated. *E. coli* can release a deadly toxin that can result in severe diarrhea, and blood vessels may be damaged enough to cause hemorrhaging.

This condition can be extremely dangerous, and possibly lethal, for small children, who cannot tolerate much blood and fluid loss. In approximately 5 to 10 percent of small children infected by *E. coli,* the illness progressed to hemolytic uremic syndrome, HUS, which is characterized by kidney failure and loss of red blood cells. In severe cases, the disease can cause permanent kidney damage.

Be assured that there are ongoing efforts to track these bugs and to prevent them from hurting us.

Should I be concerned about fish?

One should be very cautious about eating raw fish and raw shellfish—all kinds of bacteria can be present. Although almost any food may be contaminated with hepatitis virus Type A, shellfish are particularly susceptible. In fact, steaming clams may not be sufficient to kill harmful bacteria that also may be present. And, even then, you'll recall from a previous chapter that ingestion of toxins from certain harmful algae can cause paralysis. Oysters aren't immune from causing trouble, either. Eating raw oysters can be very dangerous because of the bacterium *Vibrio vulnificus* that is common to seawater. Oysters can easily become contaminated with this organism. Certain health conditions—such as liver disease, diabetes, cancer, and compromised immune systems—put people at a high risk for infection. Forty percent of those who become infected with this organism die. Its counterpart, *Vibrio parahaemolyticus,* is not as dangerous but can inflict nausea and diarrhea on unwary diners. In the face of these odds, it is hard to believe that millions of people in the United States still insist on eating raw oysters. Properly cooked oysters and clams aren't dangerous except in instances when shellfish are contaminated with the nerve-damaging chemicals produced by "red tide" algae (the dinoflagellates). In this case, heating does not harm these toxic chemicals.

How can I tell if the fish is fresh?

The FDA and the Center for Food Safety and Applied Nutrition (CFSAN) provide some answers. Here's what this organization recommends for selection of fresh fish:

- The fish's eyes should be clear and bulge a little. Only a few fish, such as walleye, have naturally cloudy eyes.
- Whole fish and fillets should have firm and shiny flesh. Dull flesh may mean the fish is old. If the flesh doesn't spring back when pressed, the fish isn't fresh.
- There should be no darkening around the edges of the fish or brown or yellowish discoloration. Fresh whole fish also should have bright red gills free from slime.
- The fish should smell fresh and mild, not fishy or ammonia-like.
- Buy only from reputable sources. Be wary, for example, of vendors selling fish out of the back of their pickup truck.
- Buy only fresh seafood that is refrigerated or properly iced.
- Do not buy cooked seafood, such as shrimp, crabs, or smoked fish, if displayed next to raw fish: Cross-contamination can occur.
- Do not buy frozen seafood if the packages are open, torn, or crushed on the edges.
- Avoid packages that are above the frost line in the store's freezer.
- If the package cover is transparent, look for signs of frost or ice crystals. This could mean that the fish has either been stored for a long time or thawed and refrozen.
- Put seafood either on ice, in the refrigerator, or in the freezer immediately after buying it. Recreational fishers who plan to eat their catch should follow

state and local government advisories about fishing areas and eating fish from certain areas.

Use these same precautions with sushi, though it is impossible to know, without performing specific tests, whether or not the raw fish is contaminated with microorganisms. There are, of course, people who enjoy sushi. However, health and nutrition experts recommend that if you are pregnant or a member of a vulnerable group previously discussed, you should not eat raw fish of any kind. The risk of contracting a food-borne illness is simply too great. Instead, select sushi that uses cooked fish and/or vegetables. If you are an otherwise normal, healthy adult and enjoy sushi, understand the risks and be familiar with the place where you eat this dish.

How do I avoid cross-contamination?

The sooner surfaces are cleaned, the better, using soap and hot water. There is no need to buy some special commercial-type or hospital-approved cleaning material for this purpose. Good old dishwashing soap,

---

In 1989, one restaurant in Missouri was associated with approximately 101 cases of *Campylobacter* infections. The infections were apparently caused when cantaloupes, pineapples, and honeydew melons became cross-contaminated after poultry and the fruit were cut on the same surfaces.

---

hot water, and a little scrubbing work just fine. Do not allow time for the bugs to grow at room temperature: Prepare the meat as quickly as you can to minimize the time at room temperature (remember that germs grow best above 40 degrees and below 140 degrees Fahrenheit).

What are the dangers surrounding eggs, cheese, and raw milk?

Each of these foods can be a source of bacterial contamination. Bacteria like *Salmonella enteriditis* can infect the ovaries of the laying hen before the shell is formed, therefore contaminating the eggs. Properly cooked or pasteurized eggs decrease the risk of infection. But one note: While the bacteria in eggs are killed when they are boiled in their shell, the process destroys much of the protection against spoilage given by the shell. Therefore, hard-boiled eggs must be refrigerated. If they are left out for more than two hours, throw them away.

Raw eggs that have not been pasteurized should not be used in recipes that will not later be cooked. Recipes that contain raw eggs, such as homemade ice cream or Caesar salads, are not considered safe. It is always best to avoid eating *any* raw eggs, which means giving up tasting raw cookie dough, no matter how delicious the thought. Do not despair: Commercially prepared cookie dough is safe—the eggs in the dough are all pasteurized.

Raw milk should also be avoided; milk should be pasteurized. Raw milk can have some vicious bugs in it, those already mentioned and a couple of others that will cause tuberculosis and brucellosis, both extremely harmful diseases. In fact, the practice of pasteurizing

> The California State Department of Health reports
> that brucellosis and other infections from eating
> unpasteurized soft cheese have occurred regularly in
> California in recent years. Because of the typical asso-
> ciation of the brucellosis cases with illegally imported
> soft cheese from Mexico, California state health offi-
> cials advised consumers to avoid cheeses sold by
> street vendors, and not to illegally transport Mexican-
> style, soft, unpasteurized cheeses into California.

milk was originally started because of the prevalence of
these two diseases.

Are there germs in cheese?

Are you kidding? Cheese would just be a puddle of
milk without bacteria. But it is the soft cheeses such as
Brie, feta, and the Mexican-style cheeses mentioned
previously that can be the most hazardous. Because
they usually harbor a significantly higher quantity of
bacteria, these cheeses have a greater probability of
containing some bad bugs.

Should I be concerned about commercially prepared canned goods?

Commercially prepared, properly canned items can
usually be stored for a very long time and are generally
safe. All canned goods should be stored in a cool, dark,

dry place. Unopened low-acid canned goods such as meat, poultry, fish, stew, soups, beans, corn, pasta, and peas may last from two to five years and retain their quality. High-acid canned foods such as juices, fruit, pickles, tomatoes, and soup may be stored anywhere from twelve to eighteen months, unopened, and will retain their quality. The industry standards and safety requirements include a heat-treatment process sufficient to kill any dangerous organism, including any spores. It is therefore an extremely rare occurrence for any of the canned goods you purchase to be a problem. However, low-acid foods, such as green beans, corn, fish, or mushrooms that have been improperly canned are the main sources of potential harm from botulism toxin.

Note: It is not a good sign when cans or containers leak, bulge, or are damaged, or when their contents spurt or foam when opened. So check cans carefully before putting them in your shopping cart. Do not open these cans—stuff could fly out, including very deadly toxins. If you happen to open something by mistake and get material on your hands, do not put your hands in your mouth or touch anything. Wash your hands really well with detergent and hot water. Clean everything carefully—using gloves—then throw everything away, including the gloves.

How about home canning?

Home canning is not as common as it was years ago, but there are many people who still enjoy canning their produce. The main concern here is spores from organisms that are present in soil. The main culprit is

Clostridium botulinum, a bacterium that can release the botulism toxin. A person need not be infected with the bacterium to be harmed by the toxin; simply ingesting the toxin is enough. But an additional soil-loving bad bug that may be involved is *Listeria monocytogenes.* Consequently, it is necessary to prepare the food properly, which means using a pressure cooker that is in good condition. In order to kill the spores that might be trapped in the produce, the pressure cooker must maintain a temperature of about 250 degrees Fahrenheit (121 degrees Celsius) for more than fifteen minutes. Sealing of the cans or jars must also be done correctly. A good idea is to contact the local USDA Extension Service office to obtain instructions on how to can foods properly.

What about leftovers?

Here is the statement found in every USDA office, in all FDA offices, and in all food-safety organizations: "If in doubt, throw it out." The general rule is that hot, cooked food should not be allowed to sit more than two hours at room temperature. If you have not eaten it or refrigerated it by then, get rid of it. And it is a good idea not to eat a dab of the food before you throw it away, no matter how tempting it seems. So do not leave food, like pizza, for example, at room temperature overnight and then chomp on it the next morning.

Generally, most cooked leftovers can be safely refrigerated at the correct temperature for three to five days. Wrappings, such as plastic wrap or foil, do not stop germs from growing. They are mainly used to keep food from drying out and to keep other odors from entering the food. When possible, though, reheat the food to the proper cooking temperature. If there is some sort of sauce like gravy or broth, only two to three days of storage is recommended. When you reheat these sauces, bring them to a boil.

You may also obtain more information from your local USDA extension office and from the FDA. Keep this kind of list handy when in the kitchen.

Cooking Temperatures

Eggs	Cook until yolks and whites are firm	
Egg dishes	160°	
Turkey, chicken	165°	
Veal, beef, lamb, pork	160°	
Beef and ground meat	Rare	145°
	Medium	160°
	Well-done	170°
Fresh lamb	Medium	160°
	Well-done	170°
Fresh pork	Medium	160°
	Well-done	170°

Cooking Temperatures *(continued)*

Poultry

Chicken, whole	180°
Turkey, whole	180°
Poultry breasts, roasts	170°
Poultry thighs, wings	180°
Stuffing (cooked alone or in bird)	165°
Duck & Goose	180°

Ham

Fresh (raw)	160°
Pre-cooked (to reheat)	140°

What is the harm in mold?

Every now and then we store food like hard cheese or jelly in the refrigerator for quite a while, only to open it and find a not-so-appetizing patch of mold. That is a sign that the item may not be safe to eat. Even if it is your great-aunt's hot pepper jelly, if you see mold, it is probably best to throw the jelly away. Some molds can produce poisons that spread into the food, jelly included.

How far the poison may have spread depends on a lot of things, so a person never knows where it is within the food. If you are like me, you are not about to break out your handy mold-detection kit and test everything. So if you cut away some mold on a piece of hard cheese or firm fruit, cut away a big piece around the mold. All in all, though, it is a better idea just to throw it out.

How long can I keep something like jelly, cheese, or peanut butter if there is no mold?

Almost everyone probably has a bottle of catsup or a jar of peanut butter that has been hanging around for a while in the fridge or on the shelf. When do these items go bad? Germs do not usually like things with lots of sugar, oil, or acid, so these items tend to last a pretty long time. Regardless of the type of purchased food, always pay attention to any "Use By Date" information on the package or item. Following are some guidelines for when you are not sure:

Unopened Food
- Hard cheese like Cheddar or Swiss can last refrigerated for about half a year.
- Soft cheeses like cream cheese should be stored only a couple of weeks in the refrigerator.
- If commercially prepared, it is not necessary to refrigerate jams or jellies if you do not open the jar. These jams and jellies will usually last up to one year if not opened and if kept in a cool, dark place.
- The same goes for mayonnaise. If produced commercially (not made at home), mayonnaise is likely good for two to three months when kept in a cool, dark place.

- And that good old standby for kids, peanut butter, can last almost nine months if the jar is closed.
- Pickles, like jellies, can last up to a year if tightly sealed.
- Bottled salad dressings will last up to one year.

Food That Is Opened and Refrigerated

- Discard hard cheeses after they have been in the refrigerator for about three weeks.
- Commercially prepared jellies in a jar will usually last up to six months.
- Mayonnaise should be chucked after two months in the fridge.
- Peanut butter can be stored in a cool, dark place on a shelf for about three months.
- Pickles ought to be discarded after one or two months.
- Salad dressings should be decent for about three months in the refrigerator. But in all of these cases, "If in doubt, throw it out!" The risk of infection simply is not worth it.

Will I glow if I eat irradiated food?

The ionizing radiation process uses gamma rays, high-energy electron beams, or X-rays to kill bacteria and inactivate viruses. The purpose of this process is to disrupt lethally the life processes of any organism that may contaminate the product. However, unless you are an astronaut in space, the irradiated food you eat will not be sterile. It will be much safer, but not sterile. This technology has actually been around for a long time and has been used specifically to protect food for more than fifty years. This procedure is supported by many professional organizations concerned with food safety, and it is known to work: Just a low-level treatment of fresh poultry can reduce germs by 99.9 percent! For the same reason that you do not become radioactive after getting a dental X-ray, you will not become radioactive if you eat irradiated food. Wheat was approved for irradiation in 1963, and by 1997 irradiation was approved for red meats (irradiation of poultry was approved in 1990). Today about forty nations irradiate food, and many, many tons are treated by this process each year.

Beyond sanitation, there are many different benefits of irradiation, not the least of which may be the reduction in chemical treatments of our food. Further, irradiation actually slows the decay process, so we can keep things fresher longer. Irradiation does not stop food from picking up germs on its way to your kitchen, though, so good food safety precautions should always be practiced.

How could fruit and vegetables be anything but healthy?

When you remove fruits and vegetables from the bags and put them on the counter, the normal assumption is that these items are fairly clean. How could something so delicious looking and nutritionally healthy *not* be clean? Well, do not be fooled; sometimes they can be hosting a ton of germs.

For example, recent studies show that bean sprouts or alfalfa sprouts may be hiding millions of *coliform* bacteria and, in particular, several thousand *E. coli* bacteria per gram (one gram is only about three-hundredths of an ounce). These bacteria, including *E. coli,* are commonly found in the intestines of animals, humans included. So their presence on food indicates that they may have been exposed to fecal material (yuck!). Although the vast majority of *coliform* bacteria will not hurt us, their presence strongly indicates that more dangerous bacteria might be present. In most cases this contamination occurs during the handling or processing of the food before or while in shipment, or after the items have arrived at the store. That is why there are such strict hygiene requirements for all those who handle, process, and/or serve food. Unfortunately, without specific tests performed in a high-tech laboratory, no one can know for sure whether or not *Shigella* or some other particularly dangerous bug is hiding among the kinder and gentler organisms.

Do contaminated fruits and vegetables occur only in certain parts of the country?

I will tell you right now that bacteria are not selective. Scientists have gone into grocery stores and markets all across the United States and randomly examined food. Their results are upsetting: Benign-looking vegetables such as radishes and cauliflower may contain thousands to millions of cells of *Listeria* and/or other potentially harmful bacteria.

What if I just wash off the germs?

Okay, so the fruit and vegetables may have a ton of germs on them. No problem, you think. Ever since you were a little kid you have been told to wash an apple before eating it. So with that in mind you grab some apples, lettuce, and tomatoes and wash them with tap water while humming a happy tune. You are confident that this flood blasts every bug from the surface and that any with the audacity to remain are either dead or unconscious.

Unfortunately, a heavy rinse does not remove, stun, or kill all germs. The ones left behind might be soaking wet, but there could be enough of them to cause a serious illness. It is not that washing does not help—it does—but these little critters can stick like glue and many cannot be washed or rubbed off.

In tests, six washes with clean water removed about 99 percent of the bacteria. Sad to say, though, that 1 percent remaining consisted of several thousand–fold more cells than is normally required to cause an illness. However, the reduction in the numbers of dangerous organisms greatly increases the chances that we will be able to handle those that remain. There is really no method yet available to remove completely all contaminating bugs from the fruit or vegetables. The best thing to do is to wash the food several times under a stream of running water to reduce the number of germs significantly. Keep in mind that it is risk reduction we are after here, not sterility.

Is there anything I can do?

If you were careful not to spread the germs to the inside of the fruit or vegetable, peeling would reduce or eliminate the number of bacteria remaining. But you know as well as I do that it is impossible to peel every piece of fruit or every vegetable that crosses our plates. When is the last time you tried to peel one of those really knobby parts of a cauliflower? By the time you got a good veggie dip ready, your guests would have gone somewhere else. So unless we cook the fruit or vegetables, we will have to accept the fact that we are likely to eat some of the little critters. Generally, though, a healthy immune system will normally fight off the germs.

Which fruits and vegetables are of special concern?

Any vegetable or fruit surface can be contaminated with potentially dangerous bacteria, as long as humans are involved in its growing, collection, and distribution. This contamination can easily be spread to the inside of the fruit when the meat inside the fruit is cut or handled. Too, the surface on which the fruit was cut can then be a source of cross-contamination of other fruits or vegetables or of anything else placed on that surface.

A growing issue nowadays is the origin of the produce—where it is grown and the initial shipping point. In 1989 there were approximately 295 cases of *Salmonella* infection (*S. chester*) traced to cantaloupes imported from Mexico. Infectious organisms will not normally be inside fruit but, as stated previously, they can most certainly be on the outside if the fruit is exposed to animal waste, contaminated water, or other sources of these bugs. So simply handling contaminated fruit or cutting it can distribute the bugs. The good news is that the United States and most other developed countries enforce strict hygiene requirements associated with food handling and distribution. These requirements significantly lower the risk of bacterial contamination in the nation's food supply. The bad news is that from time to time there are clearly holes in this net of protection. Since nobody could possibly inspect every single crate stacked in those ports, it is up to us to be cautious and to use good food safety practices.

Why is this risk particularly greater for some imported produce but not with imported meat?

Nations that do not have equivalently strict food hygiene laws are not allowed to export meat or meat products to the United States. The same regulations do not yet exist for fruit and vegetable imports. Instead, only a sampling of such goods entering our borders are inspected by the Food and Drug Administration. It is easy, then, for an unscrupulous exporter and/or importer to distribute the goods before a decision is made about the safety of the sample. After the food has been distributed, it is tough to recall everything before somebody uses it. Progress has been made on this front: In 1999 President Clinton directed agencies to hold imported produce in storage facilities until released by the FDA inspectors. Unfortunately, there are not yet enough food inspectors or storage facilities available to examine and temporarily store all of the produce that enters the United States.

So how do I go about buying imported produce?

We all know from going to the grocery store that the

food items we find there may be from almost anyplace in the world. Not all countries that supply food to the United States have the same set of strict laws about food handling as ours. Developing nations often do not have the necessary infrastructure to support adequate inspections, nor do they necessarily have the same level of sanitation requirements. Consequently, we face an increased risk of bacterial contamination when dealing with imported fresh produce from developing countries. For example, you may remember the association of illnesses caused by *Cyclospora,* a parasite similar to *Cryptosporidium,* with raspberries imported from Guatemala.

In the past, infections caused by this organism appeared only in those who traveled to a developing country. But since the increase of produce imported into the United States, this organism has been linked to illnesses here. But remember that, although there is an increased risk, it is not an absolute guarantee that you will experience a problem. So do not stop eating something packed with nutrients just because the produce is not home-grown.

How can I get more information?

All kinds of very useful information can be found to help you make good choices. One thing you can do is to ask your local grocer about the initial source of the fruit and vegetables sold and whether there are any precautions taken with respect to possible bacterial contamination. Ask specific questions and expect specific answers. One other source of good information is on the Internet, in particular the Web sites of the Food and Drug Administration (www.fda.gov) and the Centers for Disease Control and Prevention (www.cdc.gov). Also pay attention to any news articles that concern contamination. Public-health offices are very thorough about keeping track of any outbreaks, and it is a good bet that announcements will be made if there is something causing a problem in your area. You can also contact your local agricultural extension office and ask them about any local health concerns.

Because of an increased amount of illness from fruits and vegetables, plans are in the works to develop further non-toxic antibacterial sprays. One example is a mixture of vinegar and household hydrogen peroxide for distributors to use on fruits and vegetables. There are antibacterial sprays on the commercial market that can be used specifically in the home for fresh vegetables and fruit just prior to serving—check the grocery shelves for these items. Just remember that there has not yet been enough research on such products to establish their effectiveness. However, if you or someone for whom you are responsible for preparing food is a member of one of the high-risk groups, you may wish to investigate the use of such a product. Ask your physician and pharmacist for their advice.

What about "organically grown" fruits and vegetables?

Just because something is said to be "organically grown" does not necessarily make it safer. The very same risks of contamination with bacteria or viruses apply to these foods as well. As long as soil is involved and as long as humans handle and distribute the goods, contamination is always a threat. Too, fertilizer is fertilizer, whether it comes as chemicals inside a bag or in its natural state as animal waste. The difference is that animal waste contains potential disease-causing organisms. So you want to be just as careful with these kinds of produce as you are with other produce.

The one thing that might be less of an issue with "organically grown" materials is the possible absence of commercial pesticide use. However, even this issue can fool you. If a vegetable or fruit plant naturally resists insect damage, it is possible that the plant has a built-in pesticide. Insects do not leave a plant alone simply because it does not look good; they avoid it because it does not taste good. Not tasting good could possibly be due to the plant's ability to have made a powerful insecticide all on its own. This chemical could well be just as hazardous as a dose of commercial pesticide residue. That's why it is a good idea to know the producer's operation as well as possible.

How about non-pasteurized fruit juices?

Anything that is pasteurized—which includes 98 percent of all canned or bottled juices in the United States—is relatively safe. The process usually used, called flash pasteurization, heats drinks to about 162 degrees Fahrenheit—well above the growth-range maximum and into the killing zone. Once the container of pasteurized juice is opened, it should always be refrigerated. Also remember that pasteurization does not sterilize; it only eliminates the more dangerous bugs (the ones responsible for brucellosis and tuberculosis) and significantly reduces the remainder. As a consequence the food may, whether bottled or canned, spoil over time, even if it is not opened. *E. coli* O157:H7 and other microbial hazards have been related to non-pasteurized juice.

Since 1998, all non-pasteurized juices manufactured in the United States are required to have a warning label that tells you the juice has *not* been pasteurized. If you see fresh fruit juice of any kind for sale that is stored in the cold but does not have a "non-pasteurized" warning label, ask the seller about it.

In Summary

- There is always a slight risk of getting a food-borne illness whenever food is handled or prepared for eating; not only meat, but also vegetables and fruit can harbor bad bugs.
- *Campylobacter* is the leading cause of food-borne illness in the United States, with *Salmonella* second on the list.
- The sponge and dishrag are potent sources of contamination, so clean these items frequently.
- Be careful of cross-contamination. Do not use the same cutting board for meat as you do for produce, and avoid using the same utensils for food preparation as those used for serving or eating.
- Do not allow cooked food to remain at room temperature any longer than two hours before refrigeration or freezing.
- Do not thaw and then refreeze uncooked meat.

- The dishwasher water temperature should be at least 140 degrees Fahrenheit (60 degrees Celsius).
- Diluted bleach is a good disinfectant and kills bacteria and viruses.
- The refrigerator temperature should be kept between 35 and 40 degrees Fahrenheit (between about 2 and 4 degrees Celsius); the freezer temperature should be kept at 0 degrees Fahrenheit (approximately –18 degrees Celsius) or below.
- As for leftovers, "If in doubt, throw it out!"
- Unless you own a deep freeze or have a very large family or group to feed, you might think about buying in smaller quantities and replenishing more often for food freshness and food safety.

Chapter Ten

Cleaning Up Germs in the Bathroom

The bathroom is usually the first place in the home that people assume is dirty. Well, this may amaze you, but studies reveal that the bathroom is often cleaner than the kitchen. But "clean" is a relative term. There are some simple things we can do to prevent transporting germs from the bathroom to the rest of the house—and to other people.

The goal is not a perfectly sterile bathroom, because the greater the numbers of run-of-the-mill, relatively harmless bacteria that are present, the less likely it is that pathogens can find room for a decent place to live.

What is the best way to decrease the spread of infection from the bathroom?

By simply cleaning your hands after using the bathroom (an estimated 30 percent of adults do not), you can decrease the number of disease-causing germs that leave the bathroom. The important thing is that the hand-washing be fairly vigorous and last for at least twenty seconds. The friction caused by scrubbing with soap and even drying your hands helps drive the germs out of the crevices.

When these germs get down into the pores and around the oil glands, simple scrubbing will not reach them. In order for all of these bugs to be killed, much stronger hospital-grade disinfectants (that may contain iodine derivatives) and serious scrubbing would be required (surgeons, for example, are required to scrub for at least ten minutes before operating). This surgical degree of cleanliness is simply not necessary unless there is someone in the household who happens to be particularly at risk.

> Flushing the toilet can eject droplets of water, each containing thousands of germs, into the air, so close the lid before you flush.

How do soaps and detergents work?

Present-day soaps and detergents (from the Latin *detergere,* to "wipe away or off") act on dirt and excess oil to release them from surfaces and crevices of the skin—or wherever they may be. Some detergents are pretty powerful (such as Roccal) and can disinfect surfaces. Soap is made by reacting something like sodium hydroxide with vegetable oil (Dove, Pure and Natural, and Zest are a few examples). Only perfume or skin-softening agents of some sort may sometimes be added. Soap alone is not a disinfectant.

Are antibacterial soaps better than other soaps?

Interestingly, soaps containing over-the-counter germicides (antibacterials) are useful in places where people are especially prone to infection, but are often not better than regular soap for cleaning your hands. Triclorcarban, the generic name for a substance used in antibacterial soap, is very similar in structure to the generic disinfectant triclosan, which acts like an antibiotic. Soaps containing this agent claim to kill the majority of bacteria on your hands and body, but those too strong to kill are left behind. These survivors can now multiply without competition, thereby possibly increasing the chance for infection. Do not forget that it is always a matter of survival of the fittest.

While there is no evidence available yet, the overuse of these antibacterial soaps may lead to resistant strains of bacteria. Until enough tests are done, be judicious in the use of antibacterial products unless they are absolutely necessary.

Does soap kill both viruses and bacteria?

Unfortunately, there haven't been very many studies concerning the effectiveness of various regular or antibacterial soaps against viruses. What is known is that some viruses acquire a membrane after leaving a cell, and the salts of fatty acids of soap tend to disrupt the stability of this membrane. Loss of this covering will generally block the virus's ability to infect a cell. Therefore, regular hand-washing can protect us from membrane-coated viruses such as influenza and herpes.

Disease-causing viruses that do not have an envelope, such as rotavirus, Norwalk virus, and hepatitis virus Type A, can survive soap use. The chemical agents in most soap can damage the proteins exposed on the outside of these viruses, but the virus can still be infectious. As a result, it may take more than a little soap and water—perhaps some diluted bleach—to get rid of these types of viruses.

Soap seems to work really well against bacteria, including different species of *Micrococcus, Neisseria,* and *Streptococcus.* Soaps usually have sodium in them and also tend to be fairly alkaline (as opposed to acidic), both of which are harmful to bacteria. Most brands are similar and will work just fine.

> The toilet handle and the faucet handles can contain up to 50,000 bacteria per square inch.

Is the bar of soap itself clean?

Several different species of bacteria are able to live directly on the surface of bar soap. In particular, *Pseudomonas,* which can cause diseases ranging from eye infections to pneumonia, can live on the surface of bar soap, at least for a period of time. In order to lessen the chance of infection, use liquid soap dispensers throughout the house (a good idea, particularly if a person in the house has an infection of any kind). Since a person's hands do not come in contact with the soap inside the dispenser, it will not be contaminated. The dispenser itself will of course become contaminated whenever it is touched, but you will also be washing your hands immediately. Never use the bar soap directly on infected skin or on any cloth that has first contacted infected skin.

Is there any way to get rid of all of the germs?

One helpful procedure that can be used if you are particularly worried about the transfer of infection-causing organisms is to wipe everything with a solution of 70 percent alcohol (by weight), which may be purchased at your local drugstore. You can rinse your hands in it and it won't hurt you at all, but it is lethal to germs. For the alcohol to be effective you must leave the material on any surface, including your hands, for three to five minutes; do not rinse immediately. Your physician, pharmacist, or local health department will have more advice if you are especially concerned.

Should I clean the bathroom every day?

You do not need to scrub the bathroom every single day. You do, however, want to clean it thoroughly about once per week—and more often if someone in the house has diarrhea, the flu, or some infectious illness. Begin cleaning in the areas of least contamination, such as the shower, and work toward the most contaminated, in other words, the toilet (underneath the seat and the upper rim, for example). As for what kind of cleaning supplies to use, standard household soaps and detergents (without any special added ingredients) will kill many kinds of bacteria and inactivate many viruses, including the virus that causes the flu. The trick is to scrub vigorously the area you are cleaning—that is as important as anything else you can do. Remember to use diluted bleach solution for especially germy spots.

Another important way to avoid infection is to keep

hair and dirt out of the bathroom. Microorganisms latch on to such things and can contaminate us in the bargain. So vacuum and mop the bathroom floor frequently. Also be sure to clean inside, outside, and around the bottom of the toilet bowl, even under those little lids that cover the bolts at the base of the toilet and down inside where the bolt is located. Since nobody really pays attention to them (because they are somewhat scary), moisture can accumulate in these areas, creating ideal conditions for bacterial and fungal growth.

Should I throw out my sponges after cleaning the bathroom?

We have the same potential problems with the sponges used in the bathroom as we do with those we use in the kitchen: Cleaning supplies, such as sponges and brushes, are often more contaminated than the areas they are cleaning. So after every use, wash the sponges in warm, sudsy water and microwave them on full power for several minutes on high. For the brushes, soak items in the bleach solution and then rinse them out thoroughly with water. Be sure to separate the items used to clean the toilet from those items used to clean the sink, bathtub, and shower. By keeping them separate from each other, the chances of cross-contamination are very much decreased.

With all of that soap and water flying around, does the shower stay pretty clean?

To fight the growth of germs, clean the shower area

fairly often. Wiping down the shower after each use lessens moisture, thereby decreasing the growth of mold, which, beyond being an eyesore, can cause problems for people with allergies.

These critters can be removed, though, but it will take a bit of work—they are tough to kill. Use a brush of some kind and some strong bleach solution. You should use a ratio of one cup of bleach to one gallon of water. This strength of bleach solution will kill bacteria and viruses, too. It takes some time for the bleach to be fully effective, so leave the solution on whatever you are treating for ten or fifteen minutes before you rinse it away. There are some cautions that are important to remember: *Never* mix cleaning agents together or use them simultaneously to clean something without rinsing thoroughly in between the use of each, as it may cause a harmful chemical reaction. Specifically, *never* mix bleach with anything that contains ammonia because this mixture will produce hazardous fumes.

What's hiding in the towels, body sponges, and washcloths?

With respect to towels, body sponges, scrubbies, and washcloths, washing them, preferably in hot water and using chlorine bleach, kills any germs picked up in their use. Washing these items separately from the rest of the laundry is a good idea too, especially if someone in the house is ill.

Also, be careful not to leave sponges in the tub, where they will remain damp. Moisture provides a breeding ground for bacteria and fungi. To combat germ growth, either microwave the sponges or let them dry thoroughly before you reuse them.

In Summary

- The bathroom usually has fewer pathogens than the kitchen.
- Always wash your hands with soap and water after using the bathroom.
- Regular soap and water are sufficient to clean your hands if you scrub for twenty seconds or so.
- Soap alone is not a disinfectant.
- Routine use of antibacterial soaps may not be the best idea. Save these items for more serious situations like an ongoing infection in the household or for someone who may be particularly vulnerable to infections.
- Diluted bleach is a really useful disinfectant.
- Allergy-causing fungi can be killed using a fairly strong bleach solution, one cup of bleach to one gallon of water.
- *Never* mix bleach with anything that contains ammonia.
- To kill all germs, wipe everything with a solution of 70 percent alcohol (by weight), which may be purchased at your local drugstore. For the alcohol to be effective you must leave the material on any surface, including your hands, for three to five minutes.

Chapter Eleven

Where Germs Make Themselves at Home in Your Home

Besides the shoe that disappeared a couple of weeks ago, who knows what might be lurking underneath the bed? Bothersome bugs live not only underneath the bed but also in the linens, on the carpet, and all around the bedroom. In this case, some of the bugs are really bugs and the rest are our neighborhood variety of bacteria and mold spores. Let's start by taking a look at what's hiding in the dust and dander.

Should I be worried about dust devils?

Most people are not bothered too much by the dust and dander that lie about the house. However, there are lots of molds, bacteria, and a wild assortment of tiny insect and animal parts that can be found within dust. Both *Staphylococcus* and *Streptococcus* bacteria can survive in dust for months at a time. Viruses that do not have a membrane may also survive in dust for long periods, so it can easily be a source of potential infections.

Some microorganisms found in dust include:

- Fungi such as *Aspergillus* (which can cause an infection of the lungs and may also lead to asthma), *Penicillium* and *Rhizopus,* and other kinds of fungal spores
- Bacterial endospores such as those of *Clostridium* (from the same family that brings you lockjaw and botulism)
- Pollen of all kinds

There will also likely be insect fecal matter, insect parts, human skin cells, human hair, and perhaps animal hair. These items can carry bacteria on their surfaces and provide a ready source of potential infection.

While providing a common source of infectious agents, dust can also cause allergic reactions. Allergies

---

Statistics from the Centers for Disease Control and Prevention's Asthma Prevention Program:

Asthma affects more than 15 million Americans, including almost 5 million children. It is the most prevalent chronic disease among children and can be life-threatening. The death rate from asthma for children nineteen years and younger increased by 78 percent between 1980 and 1993. In 1990, costs related to asthma were estimated to total $6.2 billion; the projected cost of asthma in this country for the year 2000 is expected to double to $14.5 billion.

---

are caused whenever our bodies recognize an intruder as potentially harmful. Reactions occur when the immune system becomes activated by foreign invaders we've ingested or inhaled and begins to attack them in an inappropriate way. According to the Mayo Health Clinic, an estimated 40 to 50 percent of adults with asthma are allergic to airborne particles. As a result, we can end up with hives, swollen eyelids, a drippy nose, sneezing fits, breathing difficulties, or all of these reactions combined. If we are not careful, a serious asthma attack or other types of severe allergic reactions may lead to a hospital stay.

What can cause an allergic reaction?

Most allergic reactions stem from foreign materials in the air. Inside or outside the house, we can inhale different kinds of pollen (from grass, trees, and weeds), mold spores, small bits of animal hair (dander), or the waste and/or secretions produced by insects. If we are unlucky, we may have an allergic response to one or several of these things. Unfortunately, there is not really any absolute way to tell whether you are allergic to something except by being tested by an allergist.

Many people are allergic to bugs known as dust mites (house dust mite, or *Dermatophagoides*). These little insects are about the size of the dot over the letter "i"—you almost need a microscope to see them—and are probably the single most prevalent cause of allergies worldwide. They live all over the place, but they especially like to wiggle down inside the material of carpets, pillows, linens, mattresses, and upholstery. Do you remember in Chapter Six where we talked about how the cells of the epidermal layer of our skin die and are constantly being shed? Well, the reason we aren't wading around in several inches of dead skin cells is because dust mites eat the shed skin cells. When people with allergies test positive for house dust, more than 90 percent of the time the dust mite is the source of the allergy. When we stir things up by changing the sheets, dusting, and cleaning, the fecal matter and secretions of these little bugs fly into the air and we can inhale them. Once this material becomes lodged in the surfaces of the eye, throat, and bronchial tubes, allergic reactions can occur. So, although dust mites do us a huge favor by nibbling away at those dead skin cells, for some reason the human body doesn't take to their waste very kindly.

What can we do about this mite problem?

If you have allergies, the following are ways to reduce significantly your chance of having a reaction to dust mites.

- Completely encase the mattress, box springs, and pillows inside a plastic cover. These covers—with zippers for easy removal—can be purchased in most bed and bath stores. This cover prevents the skin cells from getting into the fabric. As a consequence of being deprived of their food, dust mites will die.
- To protect your sheets, change and wash them once a week in hot water.
- Upholstery can be a bit more of a problem, but if

the allergy is severe enough, either encase upholstered furniture in plastic or remove it from the
room. Another option is using slip-covered furniture and washing the covers regularly.

- Replace the drapes in the bedroom with plastic
shades or any nonfabric window covers.
- When you vacuum, use a cleaner with a filter in it
that will trap both the dust and the mites.
Nowadays, almost all vacuum cleaners can be purchased equipped with what is known as a HEPA
(high-efficiency particle-arresting) filter, which will
significantly cut down on particles flying around in
the air and will trap many allergy-causing particles
while we vacuum.
- For dusting, use a soft damp cloth instead of a
feather duster to lower the amount of stirred-up
dust.

How do I get those little critters out of my carpet?

Vacuuming may not be sufficient for those who have
a severe allergy to dust mites. Several products have
been developed for this purpose, but the one that seems
to work best is a diluted solution of tannic acid. This liquid, which is poisonous to the dust mite, can be sprayed
on the carpet from time to time. However, tannic acid
can be harmful to humans under certain conditions. The
old adage is true: "Sometimes the treatment can be
worse than the cure." So be sure to discuss the use of
tannic acid or any of the anti-mite products with your
allergist and pharmacist before using them to kill the
mites.

How do you reduce the number of mold spores and levels of pollen?

There are a number of relatively simple things a person can do to cut down on the amount of pollen and mold spores inside the house. When an allergy season appears (allergy seasons differ, depending on your allergy), by all means keep the windows closed whenever you can. Stay indoors in the morning, when pollen levels are at their highest. Pay attention to air quality through weather reports, which often include information on the pollen count; they often mention the number of mold spores in the air on a given day, too. You can also install a filtration barrier in your air-handling system. To minimize discomfort, change the air filters frequently on the heating and air-conditioning units according to instructions, and do not let dust and material accumulate. These preventive measures against allergies will also lower your risk of contracting respiratory illnesses from certain molds, like *Aspergillus* and *Histoplasma capsulatum*.

Will getting my air ducts cleaned help my allergies?

While the usefulness of having your home's air ducts professionally cleaned is unproven, a recent study in Texas shows the treatment is helpful. After the professional cleaning of several houses, the count of mold spores was reduced by over 90 percent. For obvious reasons, if you choose to have this service performed, first thoroughly check out the company's reputation. If your allergies are bad, cover all of the openings that vent into each room of the house with a HEPA filter and use a high-efficiency filtration device on the air-intake system.

Are there any dangers surrounding air conditioners, humidifiers, and the like?

If you place filters on the air-conditioning and heating system, the mold-spore count should remain very low. But a deadly bacterial organism, *Legionella pneumophila*, can thrive in the cooling systems. Infection by this bacterium may lead to the severe respiratory disease legionellosis. While this organism appears everywhere in our environment, it causes infection in only about 25,000 people annually in the United States. To cause an infection, this

The first known case of Legionnaires' disease caused by the bacterium *Legionella* occurred at the 1976 American Legion conference in Philadelphia, where 182 people were afflicted, 29 of whom died.

Legionnaires' disease accounts for 1 percent to 8 percent of community-acquired pneumonias that result in hospitalization. Early symptoms are similar to those of influenza: a generalized feeling of ill health accompanied by fever, muscle aches, headache, and diarrhea. Pneumonia may later develop. Legionnaires' disease may occur at any age, but most patients are middle-aged men. Identified risk factors include smoking, alcohol abuse, and immunosuppression, especially from corticosteroids.

bug, which travels in aerosols, must be inhaled into the lungs. So far, there is no evidence that the disease can be transmitted by person-to-person contact.

This organism lives best in warm temperatures with lots of moisture around, making air-conditioning evaporation towers and humidifiers ideal breeding grounds. Refrigerated air-conditioning units do not appear to be a problem, only the evaporation units that use sprayed water for cooling. While cooling systems are particularly vulnerable, this bacterium can also live in hot- and cold-water taps, and in hot-water tanks, too. To keep this bug to a minimum, regularly clean the coils of any sprayed-water evaporation units and room humidifiers with diluted bleach solution. Follow the bleach solution with clean water to flush. For home evaporation cooling units, be sure to follow the manufacturer's instructions for cleaning, or contact a reputable service to clean and maintain these units.

Is the basement as scary as it seems?

The basement, especially one that is unfinished, can be a problem source of mold growth. Because of the likely increase in cooler air—and therefore moisture—in the basement, the mold is encouraged to grow on the walls and on the floor. Lack of insulation further increases its growth, with or without dry wall (Sheetrock). So it is best if the basement is kept as warm and dry as possible. Chronic exposure to mold spores can hurt you whether or not you have an allergy.

If you have a damp basement or if flooding caused enough moisture to support the growth of mold or mildew on the walls or floor, the best thing to do is to use bleach to kill the fungus. Use about one cup per gallon of water (237 milliliters of bleach per 3.8 liters of water). Spray the bleach on all surfaces and let it soak in for at least ten minutes or so before scrubbing. Rubbing on the mildew before letting the bleach sit can cause the release of fungal spores, making it easy to inhale them.

Does the laundry room pose a special problem?

The laundry room does not harbor any unusual microorganisms except in the dust and lint generated—so vacuum inside the lint traps and behind the appliances.

The real problems can be found in the laundry itself. Because of the kinds of fabrics available nowadays, hot water is not often used to wash clothes. The lack of heat increases the chance for bacteria and viruses to survive the wash cycle. When possible, wash with bleach. Dr. Charles Gerba's study of sixty homes found that one-fifth of machines contained *E. coli*. So save all of the underwear for the last wash load and, when possible, add bleach. Every few weeks simply run bleach through a wash cycle without any clothes inside the washer, using the hot setting. This treatment will pretty much kill the viruses and bacteria that might be hanging around, especially if anyone in the house has any kind of gastrointestinal upset. In the case of illness, save that person's clothes to wash separately, which helps to lower the possibility of contamination among family members.

Are we storing any disease in the garage?

While it can sometimes seem overwhelming, it is best to keep the garage clean of dirt, dust, and debris. Mice like to live in boxes with paper in them or near any kind of pet food that might be stored in the garage. Tightly cover all food, keeping it inside a can if possible. Also, any storage rooms and closets that are not often frequented may house a mouse. If you spot mouse pellets, do not go rushing in bare-handed to remove them. Mice, their feces, and their nests can all harbor viruses.

One especially worrisome virus spread by mice is the hantavirus, which can cause a rapidly debilitating respiratory illness that can be fatal. In 1993, a series of thirty-two fatal pulmonary deaths, which occurred in the Four Corners region of the United States, were attributed to hantavirus. This emerging disease has resulted in 102 cases throughout the United States as of January 1995, at least a quarter of these resulting in death. This virus is carried by the deer mouse, which is prevalent in the southwestern United States. So be careful of any nests you spot—whether or not a deer mouse might have built it.

If you want to remove nests of any kind, spray them with a strong bleach solution (1 1/2 cups bleach to 1 gallon water) and thoroughly soak all of the material with this solution. Use disposable gloves as well as a mask containing a HEPA filter over your mouth and nose to prevent inhaling any particles that fly around as you remove the nest. Place the material in a bag, seal it, and then bag it again. If you are at all concerned about deer mice and hantavirus, ask your local USDA extension office about the prevalence in your area. You can also contact the Centers for Disease Control and Prevention in Atlanta by phone (800-311-3435) or on the Internet (www.cdc.gov) and obtain further information about this virus and how to deal with any nests.

Many wild animals wander around at night, so close the garage door before nightfall. If you notice that an animal has gained entry to your garage, you should avoid it. Do not try to capture or touch the animal. If the animal doesn't leave on its own, call the animal-control professionals in your area to get rid of it. The animal may be rabid, and a rabid animal can be particularly vicious. The rabies virus can be transmitted through saliva, but it isn't always transmitted through an animal's bite. The virus can also enter through any open area in the skin. Rabies is very dangerous; it is discussed in detail in the next chapter. If you live in a rural area without an animal control force or if you think an animal may have rabies, call the local police or sheriff and report it.

In Summary

- Dust carries an assortment of fungi, bacteria, and viruses that can put you and your family at risk for a wide variety of infectious diseases.
- Dust, dust mites, and dander also cause allergic reactions in many adults and children, often resulting in a chronic respiratory condition known as asthma.
- Some things you can do to allergy-proof your home include frequently vacuuming with a cleaner

equipped with a HEPA filter, encasing upholstered furniture in plastic, and replacing drapes or curtains with plastic shades.

- Preventive measures for allergy sufferers include installing a filtration barrier in your air-handling system, keeping windows closed and staying indoors when the pollen count is high, and having your home's air ducts professionally cleaned.
- In order to cut down on the risk of contaminating your laundry, run bleach every few weeks through one hot-water wash cycle without clothes to kill any germs that may be hanging around in your washing machine.
- Remember to keep the garage clean and relatively free of dust, dirt, and debris to avoid attracting mice, which carry bacteria and viruses. One of the most dangerous viruses you can contract from the feces and nests of mice is the emerging hantavirus, which can be fatal.
- Contact the Centers for Disease Control and Prevention in Atlanta by phone (800-311-3435) or on the Internet (www.cdc.gov) to obtain further information about the hantavirus and how to deal with any mice nests.
- Actively avoid any kind of direct contact or confrontation with a wild animal, as it may be infected with the rabies virus. If you see a wild animal lurking around your home, call the animal-control professionals in your area to handle it.

Chapter Twelve

With Friends Like These—Pets and Other Creatures

Pets give us the greatest gift perhaps any friend can give: the gift of unconditional love. But these furry friends can sometimes give us other gifts we could probably do without. In addition to infectious diseases, anyone with an allergy knows of the constant battle with the dander generated by the ever-shedding dog, cat, or bird.

But hair isn't the only thing that can be flying around these and other pets. We need to watch out for what microorganisms they might harbor, too. Dogs, cats, birds, and reptiles may carry viruses and bacteria that can be very harmful to us. If we get a disease from an animal, the disease is a called a zoonosis. Some of these germs are dangerous to all humans, while others are more dangerous to people with special health concerns. Because of this danger and for general health reasons, have your pet routinely examined by a veterinarian—preventative health care is as good for them as it is for us.

If my dog licks me, will I be sickened by my dog's germs?

Contrary to how Lucy felt about Snoopy's kisses, it is probably better for you to be licked by a dog than for a dog to be licked by you. A dog's mouth is fairly acidic and not all that hospitable to pathogenic germs. So do not worry too much if the dog sneaks in a lick or two—you will survive. You might have heard of the old wives' tale that suggests a dog's lick will help heal wounds. Even though a dog's lick might not be chock-full of bad germs and seems to work well on the dog's scrapes, for humans an antiseptic ointment and a bandage act as better treatments.

Can I have a pool party with my pooch?

Having fun with your dog is one thing, but it is best to avoid swimming with him. (Cats might be a problem too, but, unlike dogs, most cats really hate doing laps in the pool.) The problem with swimming with the dog is the bacterium *Leptospira interrogans:* This bacterium can infect dogs (as well as rodents and wild animals), settling in the dog's kidneys without causing the dog to exhibit any particular symptoms. The urine of the dog may contain this bacterium, and if you swallow water with the bacterium in it or have an open place in your skin, you could get the infection. It is more common in tropical and temperate regions of the world.

Leptospirosis can cause a wide range of symptoms in humans, from high fever, severe headache, chills, muscle aches, and vomiting to none at all. Sometimes there is liver dysfunction and one might become jaundiced (as evidenced by yellow skin and eyes). Too, one can experience red eyes, abdominal pain, diarrhea, or a rash. If the disease is not treated, kidney damage, meningitis (inflammation of the membranes around the brain and spinal cord), liver failure, and respiratory distress can occur. In rare cases death occurs.

If you clean up a dog's "mistake," make sure your hands are not exposed to the dog's urine, because these bacteria can also get into our system through any little abrasion you might have on your hands.

What microorganisms do fleas and ticks carry?

Keep your animal free of fleas and ticks. Diseases like Rocky Mountain spotted fever, caused by the bacterium *Rikettsia rikettsii,* can be acquired as a result of a tick bite. The bacteria can live inside the tick and can be transmitted to you via the dog. If you live in a rural area, it is harder to prevent ticks from associating with your pet, but try to keep them off the animal as best you can.

There are some very good anti-tick and anti-flea products available. Some act systemically and are given by placing a liquid preparation on the animal's skin. Others involve bathing the animal. Talk with your veterinarian about the best product for your particular animal.

What about the bugs I get from bugs?

Ticks can infect you with germs that can cause several life-threatening diseases. The most common is Lyme disease, which was first identified in the United States around 1975. At that time, there was a puzzling and significant increase in the number of juvenile rheumatoid arthritis cases diagnosed among children in and around the town of Lyme, Connecticut. Upon investigation, Lyme disease was found to be caused by bites from ticks infected with the bacterium *Borrelia burgdorferi*. Present in the United States, Europe, and Asia, the bacterium is carried by a couple of different kinds of ticks, but the most common is the deer tick. While on average only about 1 percent of all deer ticks carry this bacterium, in some areas over 50 percent of the ticks can have it. If the disease isn't detected relatively early and is left untreated by antibiotic therapy, it can lead to some very serious maladies.

Lyme disease is not the only thing a person can get from a tick bite. Ticks can spread a form of encephalitis (inflammation of the brain), as well as a disease emerging in the United States but already present elsewhere in the world known as ehrlichiosis, which is caused by the

From the CDC: Over the past ten years, 90 percent of all reported cases of Lyme disease have occurred in the following states: New York, 39,370; Connecticut, 17,728; Pennsylvania, 14,870; New Jersey, 13,428; Wisconsin, 4,760; Rhode Island, 3,717; Maryland, 3,410; Massachusetts, 2,712; Minnesota, 1,745; Delaware, 1,003. Lyme disease is endemic in large areas of Asia and Europe.

germs known as *Ehrlichia chaffeensis, E. equi, E. phago-cytophila,* and *E. ewingii.* Since these organisms and the diseases they cause are also present in other countries in the world, your best bet is to avoid tick-infested areas, no matter where you may travel.

How can I avoid ticks, and, if I cannot, how can I get rid of them?

Wherever there are wild animals, there will be ticks. Heck, you can even get them mowing your lawn, but they are most often picked up walking in brush or tall grass. When hiking, you'll be exposed to ticks pretty much everywhere except in the dirt in the middle of a trail, and they are most prevalent during the warmer months of the spring and summer.

If you plan to be somewhere where ticks are located, the suggestions to protect you include:

- Walk in the middle of trails
- Wear light-colored, long-sleeved shirts and long pants. Tuck your pants into your socks and, preferably, wear boots that have a high top
- Wear a hat
- Use insect repellent

From time to time on your outing, check for ticks on your clothing. If you see them, remove them. Immediately after you return from your trek, take off all of your clothes and either check yourself or have someone check you from head to toe. If children are with you, check for them. If you have a pet with you, check your pet, too. Ticks like to hang around warm places and where there is some body hair, but they'll also latch on to your ankle.

To remove a tick, use tweezers and push down on the skin nearby while gently grasping the tick—do not squeeze it. Gently tug until the tick loosens its hold, then pull it off and kill it. Since it usually takes several hours for the tick to transmit its germs to you, the sooner you remove the tick, the better off you are.

Are mosquitoes dangerous or just annoying?

If you are like me, you have spent half your summer scratching mosquito bites, which are actually caused by an allergic reaction to the mosquito's saliva. But a more serious consequence of some mosquito bites may be transmission of certain serious diseases such as malaria, dengue fever, and several forms of encephalitis. Not only can mosquitoes carry diseases that afflict humans, they also can transmit several diseases and parasites that infect dogs and horses, including dog heartworms and eastern equine encephalitis.

Malaria is common in most tropical and subtropical countries, especially Central and South America, the Caribbean, sub-Saharan Africa, India, Southeast Asia, the Middle East, and the South Pacific. For every 1 million people traveling to developing countries for a one-month stay, about 24,000 would develop malaria if visiting West Africa, while 500 would if visiting South America. Commonly characterized by fever, chills, headache, and sweating, the disease may cause relapses throughout an infected person's life. Malaria caused by *Plasmodium falciparum,* the most serious form of malaria, may progress to organ failure, coma, or even death.

Dengue is a viral illness spread by mosquitoes. The occurrence of dengue fever has been spreading rapidly over the past twenty years, with millions of cases occurring each year. The risk of dengue is greatest in tropical countries of the Indian subcontinent, Southeast Asia, southern China, Central and South America, the Caribbean (including Puerto Rico and the U.S. Virgin Islands), Mexico, and Africa. The symptoms of dengue may resemble those of influenza and may last up to ten days, but complete recovery may take up to four weeks. A severe fatal form of the disease called dengue hemorrhagic fever can also occur, especially in children under age fifteen.

Encephalitis is an infection of the brain that can be caused by viruses and bacteria, including viruses transmitted by mosquitoes. West Nile encephalitis is an infection of the brain caused by West Nile virus, a flavivirus commonly found in Africa, west Asia, Eastern Europe, and the Middle East. It is closely related to the St. Louis encephalitis virus found in the United States.

Your best protection against any mosquito-borne illness is to use precautions such as mosquito netting and to apply an insect repellent while outdoors. The most effective repellents are those that contain at least a 20 to 30 percent concentration of DEET.

I wouldn't hurt a flea, but can a flea hurt me?

Fleas can carry disease, especially in the western part of the United States, or the continents of Africa, Asia, or South America. The Black Death that ravaged Europe in the Middle Ages, also known as the plague, is caused by the bacterium *Yersinia pestis* that fleas carry. The fleas pick up the disease from wild animals—such as rats, ground squirrels, and gophers—and transmit it to you. So do not feed or handle any of these wild animals, and do not generate conditions that will attract them. Also make sure any pets you have with you are treated with anti-flea medication.

Can dry cat or dog food that is left out in the open spoil?

Since most packaged dry dog or cat food is made with preservative agents, such as ascorbic acid and BHA, it is relatively safe to leave out for an entire day without worrying about it becoming contaminated. However, if the conditions of the room where the food is stored are especially moist, or if the food is left out for more than one day, bacterial or fungal growth can occur. If you buy dry pet food in bulk, it is best to buy in relatively small quantities and store food in an airtight container.

Are cats cleaner than dogs?

On the surface, cats appear much cleaner than dogs; they are certainly more fastidious when it comes to washing themselves. The common household cat, however, can be a significant source of infections. One disease, commonly known as cat-scratch disease (although dogs can harbor this bacterium too), is caused by the bacterium *Bartonella henselae*. Animals do not usually show any evidence of being infected by the bacteria, so your cat (or dog) needs to be periodically tested. If you do get the disease and you are relatively healthy, it will usually resolve on its own in about six to twelve weeks. Some symptoms of cat-scratch disease include swollen lymph nodes (in the neck and groin), perhaps a fever, tiredness, and sometimes vomiting. There can also be a headache, a sore throat, and weight loss. In some people there will be an obvious infection at the site of the scratch itself.

Cat-scratch disease is not particularly harmful to humans, unless a weak immune system is involved. However, another disease known as *Bacillary angiomatosis,* which is characterized by sequestration of the bacteria in pockets underneath the skin and by broken blood vessels underneath the skin (professionally termed cutaneous and subcutaneous vascular lesions), has also been associated with this bacterium.

As the name implies, scratches from a cat (or a dog, less commonly) are the causes of infection. To avoid this one, try to keep roughhousing to a minimum. If an animal does scratch you, clean the wound as soon as possible with soap and water or hydrogen peroxide solution. If your immune system is weak, tell your physician about the scratch—then watch the scratch closely and pay attention to any symptoms that may appear.

Don't Touch That Doorknob!

Do cats pose a special threat to pregnant women?

Another disease one can contract from cats, toxoplasmosis, is particularly dangerous to the unborn fetus of a pregnant woman and persons with substantially weakened immune responses. The disease is caused by a single-cell parasite named *Toxoplasma gondii* that is often found in cat feces. The Centers for Disease Control and Prevention states that "more than 60 million people in the United States are probably infected with the *Toxoplasma* parasite, but very few have symptoms because the immune system usually keeps the parasite from causing illness."

Babies born to mothers who are *first* exposed to *Toxoplasma* infection several months before or *during* pregnancy are at risk for severe disease. However, many exposed infants have no symptoms at all. The unborn child can become permanently mentally and physically harmed if the mother becomes infected with this parasite. Thus, a pregnant woman should avoid emptying cat-litter boxes until after the baby is born. Digging around barehanded in the flowerbeds or garden—places cats like to frequent—isn't a good idea, either. If you are worried about this organism, have both yourself and your cat tested for infection.

Do I need to worry about rabies?

We do not hear much about people contracting rabies anymore, but the disease caused by this virus is so dangerous that it is a good idea to know about the symptoms. The rabies virus is extremely harmful, and all

180

warm-blooded animals are susceptible to infection—including humans. In 1997, in the United States there were 8,500 cases of rabies in animals and four cases in humans reported to the Centers for Disease Control and Prevention. The virus is usually transmitted by saliva through bite wounds, and without proper treatment it can cause a terrible neurological disease that can be fatal. However, if immunization is given within two days of the bite, rabies is usually prevented. Once the symptoms appear, few people survive the disease. Death from respiratory failure usually occurs within seven days. In 1940 or so, domestic animals, dogs in particular, were recognized to be the most common carrier for the rabies virus in the United States. Efforts were subsequently made to vaccinate all dogs and cats in the United States against this virus.

Since this long-standing vaccination program has been in effect, the incidence of rabies in domestic animals has dropped dramatically. Unfortunately, in wild animals the rate of infection has increased. Although skunks, bats, and foxes are prone to infection, the raccoon is now thought to be the leading carrier of the rabies virus in wild-animal populations. An intelligent animal, the raccoon is very curious and may visit your yard to take a look around or to search for food and water. Even wooded suburban areas may have this rascal out and about (or sometimes in the attic), so take care to stay away from it.

If your pets venture outside on their own they might run into a rabid animal, so it is best to keep your pets close to home. Do not allow them to come in contact with what might appear to you to be a stray pet—even if your own pet is vaccinated against rabies. If you see an animal that looks disoriented or particularly aggressive, leave it alone. If the animal appears injured but you did not see the injury occur, do not try to help the animal or even approach it. Instead, contact an animal control officer or the sheriff.

What microorganisms flock to our fine feathered friends?

Birds can harbor some creepy germs. Birds (particularly poultry) can carry *Campylobacter fetus* or *Campylobacter jejuni*. Both of these bacteria can cause mild to severe cases of diarrhea—and youngsters and the elderly may have a more difficult time with it. In the last several years, these bacteria have been identified to be the leading cause of diarrhea in the United States.

While we normally contract this organism via contaminated food (especially poultry) or water, we can also be infected through our pet bird, dog, or cat. While birds are not the only pets that may harbor these bacteria, cleaning their cages or pens may make the bird owners especially vulnerable. If you have birds for pets, try not to allow their droppings to become dry. Dried feces and urine can enter the air as small particles as the birds flap around in the cage or as you clean the cage. These particles in the air, called aerosols, can be easily inhaled.

So clean the bird's cage frequently, and remember to double-bag the waste material. Do not store the waste for a long time before disposal—as it can dry out and generate aerosols when the bags are moved

From the CDC: "Most people who get *campylobacteriosis* recover completely within two to five days, although sometimes recovery can take up to ten days. In rare cases, some long-term consequences can result from a *Campylobacter* infection: Some people may have arthritis following *campylobacteriosis*; others may develop a rare disease that affects the nerves of the body beginning several weeks after the diarrheal illness. This disease, called Guillain-Barré syndrome, occurs when a person's immune system is triggered to attack the body's own nerves, which can lead to paralysis that lasts several weeks and usually requires intensive care. Approximately one in every 1,000 reported *campylobacteriosis* cases leads to Guillain-Barré syndrome, and as many as 40 percent of the cases in this country may be triggered by *campylobacteriosis*."

around. Make sure that you check with your veterinarian and have the birds examined annually for any sign of disease.

Parrots and parakeets are also especially prone to carrying the bug *Chlamydia psittaci*, which causes parrot fever, or psittacosis. Turkeys are good sources of this organism too. Not only bird owners or commercial suppliers of such pets, but also those who are involved in commercial operations with birds, like turkeys, should be aware of this disease. So again, if you clean the cage often and completely, thoroughly wash your hands. Each cleaning prevents particles of fecal material and

From the New York City Department of Health, Bureau of Communicable Disease: "Current laws require that members of the parrot family that are imported from foreign countries be kept in a bird quarantine station prior to sale. During the quarantine, they are given feed containing tetracycline to reduce the risk of infection, but the duration of treatment is generally shorter than the 45 days necessary to completely treat the bird. Therefore, federal health authorities have recently recommended that breeders and importers ensure that all domestic nestlings and imported birds receive the special tetracycline feed for 45 continuous days in order to prevent the spread of *psittacosis* from birds to humans."

urine from accumulating and infiltrating the air you breathe.

What about wild birds?

Wild birds can also be a breeding ground for infectious organisms. Occasionally, the organism that causes parrot fever can be found in pigeons, so avoid handling them. Unfortunately, there are quite a few other organisms that can hop from birds onto humans: the bacterium *Mycobacterium avium,* which causes a kind of tuberculosis; the fungus *Histoplasma capsulatum,* which is responsible for another kind of lung disease known as histoplasmosis, caused by inhaling the spores. So stay away from large concentrations of wild birds, and especially from the soil underneath where they roost and leave their droppings. Also avoid handling bird nests because they can release the dander and dried feces into the air.

Do birds carry the West Nile virus?

The West Nile virus is indeed capable of infecting birds, as well as humans. West Nile virus was first recognized in the Western Hemisphere in 1999, when a case of encephalitis, later traced to this virus, appeared in New York City. This virus was found to have killed a number of American crows in the area, but this same effect on other wild birds has not been reported. According to the CDC, the disease is most commonly

---

The CDC states that "West Nile encephalitis is an infection of the brain caused by West Nile virus, a flavivirus commonly found in Africa, West Asia, and the Middle East. It is closely related to St. Louis encephalitis virus found in the United States. It is not known how long it has been in the U.S., but CDC scientists believe the virus has probably been in the eastern U.S. since the early summer of 1999, possibly longer. Prior to August 1999, West Nile virus had never been reported in the U.S. In 1999, 61 cases of severe disease and 7 deaths occurred in the New York (metropolitan) area." According to the CDC and USDA investigations of the incident, this virus was also responsible for the deaths of several horses on Long Island, New York.

---

transmitted by the bite of mosquitoes, not by infected birds. Still, it is never a good idea to handle a wild animal of any kind bare-handed.

The virus gathers in the salivary glands of mosquitoes that feed on infected birds. If a mosquito that is carrying the virus later bites you, the virus will be transmitted into the bloodstream and you may contract the illness. Dogs and cats (horses too), if bitten by these mosquitoes, may also become infected with the virus. Most infections in humans are mild, and symptoms include fever, headache, and body aches, often with skin rash and swollen lymph glands. More severe infection may be marked by headache, high fever, neck stiffness, stupor, disorientation, coma, tremors, convulsions, muscle weakness, paralysis, and, rarely, death.

There is no particular therapeutic treatment for pets or humans that will kill the virus; they and we depend on the immune system. In serious cases, hospitalization may be required to reduce the effects of the illness while the body gets rid of the virus. There is no evidence that this virus can be transmitted from animal to human (or vice versa), from animal to animal, or from human to human. Were it not for those darn mosquitoes, we likely wouldn't need to worry at all. So, to block the spread of this and other encephalitis viruses, efforts are made to rid an area of these pests. However, there are some things you can do to protect yourself:

- Stay indoors at dawn, at dusk, and in the early evening.
- Wear long-sleeved shirts and long pants whenever you are outdoors.

- Apply insect repellent sparingly to exposed skin. An effective repellent will contain 35 percent DEET (N,N-diethyl-meta-toluamide). DEET in high concentrations (greater than 35 percent) provides no additional protection and may be harmful.
- Repellents may irritate the eyes and mouth, so avoid applying repellent to the hands of children.
- Spray clothing with repellents containing permethrin or DEET, as mosquitoes may bite through thin clothing.
- Whenever you use an insecticide or insect repellent, be sure to read and follow the manufacturer's directions for use, as printed on the product.

You may think that mosquitoes can also transmit the flu to humans, but they cannot. Although both domestic and wild birds can be infected with various strains of influenza virus Type A (the source of such flu epidemics as the "Hong Kong" and "swine" flu in humans), mosquitoes are not involved in transmission of the flu virus. Unlike the West Nile virus, the influenza virus cannot live inside a mosquito. We can become infected with the flu simply by being in close contact with such birds, much as we can become infected with the flu virus by being in close contact with a human who has the flu.

Can you catch a cold from cold-blooded reptiles?

An estimated 7 million reptiles are kept as pets in the United States alone. Although I never owned one as a pet, as a child I enjoyed watching little green chameleons play around in the ferns kept on the front porch. As it turns out, I'm probably lucky they were too fast to catch; I did not know at the time what germs these lizards might be carrying around with them.

The major health issue concerning contact with both domesticated and wild reptiles is the *Salmonella* virus. While the most common route for infection is contaminated water or food, this bacterium can also enter the body through any open wound, no matter how tiny. This bacterium can be transferred directly from animal to animal and from human to human, and indirectly to another human by someone who has handled an infected animal. So, even though one person might not become infected, that person nevertheless may transfer the bug to someone who can then become infected. With this in mind, there should never be a reptile of any kind kept as a pet in a place of day care or in a pre-school classroom because children younger than eight are particularly susceptible to these germs.

Most reptiles do not breed well in a crowded environment. Therefore, most are not bred and raised in captivity (where their environment can be controlled) but are caught in the wild and later shipped to their destination. This practice greatly increases the chance that *Salmonella* will be riding along inside the animal's intestines. In fact, this bacterium is essentially endemic in reptiles, which means that no matter where the reptile originated, this bacterium likely came along for the ride. The common presence of *Salmonella* in reptiles is similar to the common presence of *E. coli* in humans. Because of the existence of the bug inside the reptile's intestines, this bacterium is shed in the fecal matter of the reptile. Since reptiles for the most part like water around and about them, the bacteria can contaminate all kinds of surfaces and us if we are not careful.

Many people wash their pet reptiles or let them play around in the bathtub, bathroom sink, kitchen sink, or even the shower. While it may look cute to see Tommy the turtle paddling around in the bathtub with your five-year-old, actually it is dangerous. And, unless you thoroughly wash and disinfect the surfaces of the sinks, bathtub, or shower where the reptile has traveled, germs can later easily be transferred to somebody else. So keep any kind of container that the reptile has been inside separate from all other containers. The same goes for anything used to clean the reptile's abode or feeding dishes. Never wash the pet near any glasses, toothbrushes, dishes, or utensils of any kind or they may become contaminated. Wear rubber gloves and then wash your hands when you are finished cleaning that scaly critter. Check with your veterinarian and pharmacist and find out what kind of disinfectants you should use to protect yourself. And do not forget the old bleach solution we've talked about—germs really do not like it.

The Centers for Disease Control and Prevention states, "Every year approximately 40,000 cases of *Salmonellosis* are reported in the United States. Because many milder cases are not diagnosed or reported, the actual number may be twenty or thirty times greater. It is estimated that approximately 1,000 persons die each year with acute *Salmonellosis*."

However, neither do frogs. So make sure all of the bleach is thoroughly rinsed away before the iguana crawls back into his personal sauna.

In Summary

- Pets, like humans, need regular checkups by a professional.
- Pets can be a source of human allergic reactions. Reactions against hair or feathers can sometimes be serious and should not be ignored.
- Pets can be a source of human disease–causing bacteria and viruses.
- Do not swim or bathe with your dog.
- Do not let the cat scratch you.
- Store pet food in a closed container, protecting both you and your pet from the bugs you can and can't see.
- It is usually okay if your dog licks you, but do not lick your dog.
- To protect the fetus, pregnant women should not handle soiled cat litter because of the risk of contracting toxoplasmosis.
- *Campylobacter* is a concern with pet birds—this bacterium is the leading cause of gastrointestinal illness in the United States.
- Reptiles generally carry *Salmonella* as a natural inhabitant of their intestines. This organism can sometimes cause severe illness.
- Children, some say up to age eight, should not handle reptiles of any kind, including turtles.

- Fleas and ticks can carry dangerous diseases, such as bubonic plague and Lyme disease.
- Rabies is a terrible disease. Make certain that your pet is immunized against it.
- West Nile encephalitis is an infection of the brain caused by West Nile virus that is commonly transmitted by the bite of the mosquito.

Chapter Thirteen

Dining Out with Uninvited Guests

Who does not enjoy occasionally eating out at a restaurant? And sometimes it is really convenient to stop on our way home at a deli or salad bar to buy a dinner. The family picnic, the church social gathering, and the fund-raising pancake breakfast can all be a wonderfully fun eating experience. But if these meals are prepared improperly, they will make you wish you had stayed home and eaten dry cereal from the box.

Whenever we eat food prepared by someone else, what we do not know about the food can expose us to a risk of bacterial contamination. Generally, young, healthy people who run across contaminated food may suffer a fair amount of discomfort but rarely any long-term consequences. However, it is important for seniors and those with compromised immune systems to be more cautious.

From 1993 through 1997, over 2,700 outbreaks of food-borne illness in the United States were reported to the CDC, resulting in more than 86,000 illnesses. In an article from the journal *Emerging Infectious Diseases*, Janet E. Collins of the American Meat Institute wrote,

"Recent data indicate that 80 percent of reported food-borne illness outbreaks occur outside the home."

The FDA imposes the standards for restaurant safety on state and local jurisdictions. The Food Code, which is updated every two years, includes temperatures for cooking, cooling, refrigeration, reheating, and holding food in food-service establishments. County or city employees are generally charged with responsibility for inspecting restaurants; each state or locality has its own laws governing restaurant safety.

Although no nationwide mandate currently exists, additional standards imposed by states, counties, or cities can require certified training in food safety of food-service personnel, in particular the food manager of the establishment. However, only a small number of states and cities have this mandate, including California, Florida, Mississippi, and Louisiana. In some instances, even though there is no overall state mandate for certification, counties or cities within a state may require certification of food-service managers. For example, major cities such as New York City, Kansas City, and Oklahoma City have such a mandate even though the state as a whole does not require such certification. But even with restaurant inspections and, in some cases, the presence of personnel trained in food safety in the restaurant, you still need to be careful when eating out.

Are some foods more risky than others?

Some foods are higher risk than others in regard to their disease-carrying potential: Foods such as non-pasteurized fruit juices, rare or medium-rare ground meat like beef (hamburger) or turkey, raw unpasteurized eggs or eggs that aren't cooked sufficiently, raw alfalfa or other sprouts, and raw shellfish, particularly oysters, are more likely to cause you harm than other foods. If you are uncertain about the contents of a dish, do not hesitate to ask about the ingredients.

Even if the personnel at a restaurant are conscientious about safe food handling and preparation, there is always a certain amount of risk that a particular food item contains a virus or bacterium that might make us ill. To estimate the risk further, also ask how the food is prepared. For example, the dressing for a Caesar salad or a dish of homemade ice cream may contain raw eggs. If eating at a restaurant, by all means ask your waiter or waitress if these items are commercially prepared or made in-house. If they are made in-house, ask if the chef uses raw or pasteurized eggs. If raw eggs are used, it is probably best to avoid the sauce or dressing. If the ice cream is homemade, make sure pasteurized eggs were used, which are now available in the shell. These eggs will be a bit more costly but will be safer to use.

What steps are taken by restaurants to insure that I do not get sick?

A well-run restaurant will know how to prepare food correctly and the quality control will normally be pretty high. Also, given the fact that word-of-mouth reviews are passed among patrons, restaurants have a natural pressure to be careful. Besides protecting their reputation, restaurants have to follow professional regulations that are mandated by federal, state, and local governments in regard to food safety. Therefore, a fair amount of routine inspections occur in restaurants or at other public eating establishments.

What can I look for to help me know a restaurant or buffet is reasonably safe?

Of course, one of the easiest things to do is to know the place you frequent.

- The bathrooms are often a good indication of the overall cleanliness of an establishment. Are they clean and well kept? If these rooms seem to be well maintained, chances are the same hygienic standards will be found in the kitchen. Similarly, if these rooms are not clean, there is a possibility that other parts of the establishment are similarly ignored.
- Look at the table, the dining room, and the dishes and utensils to see if they are clean. If one or more of these items look dirty to you, that is not a good sign—the kitchen may be equally dirty.
- Is the food served to you piping hot? If what is supposed to be hot food is served warm, it points not only to poor management but also to possible bacterial contamination. Ask the server please to re-heat the food—simply do not accept it otherwise.
- If the food servers have any contact with your food, they should be wearing gloves and have their hair covered.

Use common sense and feel comfortable asking management any questions if you have concerns.

If a buffet is prepared for a gathering or served in a public eating place, food can be risky to eat if it is not prepared and set up properly. Any cooked food that remains between the danger zone of 40 and 140 degrees Fahrenheit for two or more hours has an increased potential to be unsafe. If you are going to a friend's party and arrive late, it is probably not a good idea to eat any food that has been sitting out for a couple of hours at room temperature. The risk is not enormous, but any germs that were not killed when the food was cooked can multiply rapidly once the temperature cools.

If the buffet is at a hotel, a restaurant, or the like, check to see if the hot food is actually kept hot—at least 140 degrees Fahrenheit. In many such places you will see a thermometer inside the dish. Check to see if the hot food container is heated continuously, and if the food is replaced in a timely manner. The busier the buffet is, the more likely that the food is turned over rapidly and is therefore less risky to eat.

Restaurant Business, June 10, 1995, states that improper hand-washing of food-service workers is thought to be responsible for approximately 12.5 million cases of food-borne illness each year in the United States.

What kinds of regulations are in place to keep me safe?

The state and county health departments examine food establishments and follow strict guidelines in regard to maintenance of food safety. Infractions are regarded as either non-critical or critical. Each infraction is counted as a negative score and the final tally is subtracted from 100 to yield the final score. Each non-critical infraction unrelated to food safety, such as a rusty bolt or a displaced tile, may count as only one point against the establishment. Critical violations, such as a dishwasher's water temperature being too low, may result in more than a five-point deduction. You can ask to see the inspection results that are supposed to be displayed in some reasonably prominent place.

Unfortunately, because of the lack of health inspectors, most cities and states simply cannot inspect every single bar, restaurant, deli, or cafeteria frequently. For example, New York state alone has approximately 28,000 delis and supermarkets that require health inspections—and only seventy-five inspectors to do the work. You do not need to be a math genius to figure out that, on average, each inspector is responsible for more places than there are days in the year. As a result, it is very important to be wary and informed, especially if you are a member of those vulnerable groups discussed in earlier chapters who should be especially concerned about food contamination.

So if you have a favorite deli, salad bar, or restaurant (including fast-food establishments), for starters read the results of the most recent health-inspection report and by all means check the report's date. If the establishment hasn't been visited since 1954, you might be in the wrong place to eat.

What about leftovers in those doggie bags?

If you are going to eat food or refrigerate it before two hours have passed since you were served, the risk of a food-borne illness is slight. If you cannot, leave your leftovers at the restaurant. The inside of the car can get pretty warm, and if the food is between 40 and 140 degrees, it can quickly become contaminated. Once you arrive home, refrigerate the leftovers immediately. When you are ready to eat the leftovers, re-heat the food to 165 degrees Fahrenheit to kill any germs that may have taken hold. If you order take-out and do not want to eat it immediately, make sure to keep the food in the oven at 160 degrees Fahrenheit until you are ready to serve it. If you bring cold food home and do not intend to eat it right away, store the food in the refrigerator just as you would any purchased cold item.

What are the dangers in food from delis and salad bars?

Most organisms that make food spoil—such as different species among the bacteria *Lactobacillus, Serratia, Erwinia, Citrobacter,* and *Leuconostoc*—are not the same bacteria that make us sick. Remember our discussion in Chapter Nine about cooked and raw food in the home and possible bacterial contamination? Well, the same holds true for salad bars and delis. The two-hour time limit for food at room temperature or warmer before discarding and/or replacing holds true for these places, as most bacteria grow like crazy between 40 degrees and 140 degrees Fahrenheit. People who work at a deli or who maintain a salad bar should replace the food—meaning *all* of the food in the container—that has been kept at room temperature for more than two hours. If they do not, there is a substantially increased risk that we may acquire a food-borne illness from that food.

We do, however, have to depend on good management as well. Make sure the people who prepare the salad bar or hot-food buffet do not add newly prepared food on top of older food. The entire contents should be replaced about every two hours if the food is kept warm—and not by scraping the leftovers out of the old container, but by completely replacing containers. Cold food should be kept on ice or refrigerated. If the lettuce looks wilted and the cauliflower sections are leathery enough to cobble shoes, somebody is waiting too long to replace things. Ask the manager—and insist on straight answers—if leftover food is kept overnight and used the following day to mix with the freshly prepared food. If so, consider frequenting a different place.

Also, be aware of those with direct contact with food: If you see personnel handle containers or food items with bare hands, watch out. Bacteria, as well as viruses, can be easily transferred from the server's hand to the food. By the same token, if the person in line in front of you decides to grab a couple of olives with his or her fingers, avoid taking any of the remaining olives and ask somebody to replace the entire bunch. Do not let your children touch vegetables at the salad bar or handle the business end of the tongs or implements (I'm assuming that you are old enough to know better than to do such a thing yourself). Obviously, if you see somebody sneeze into the lettuce, it might be a good idea to avoid it.

And what is the last thing you often do before sitting down to a deli meal?

Pay with germ-laden money, of course. While you would think currency would be brimming with disease-causing germs, metal coins and paper bills are generally too dry to support bacteria, states Michael Norgard, Ph.D., a microbiologist at the University of Texas Southwestern Medical Center. But bacteria or viruses on your hands can transfer to the money when you hand it over and therefore to the person who takes the money. If the person who takes the money also prepares your meals, make sure that he or she either puts gloves on or washes his or her hands before handling the food.

How can I possibly refuse to eat Aunt Sally's potato salad?

Despite the fact that restaurants, cafeterias, and fast-food joints can sometimes be risky, you can become as ill from Uncle Joe's chicken salad at the family reunion as you can from eating lunch at the local burger joint.

With family and friends, we are afraid to hurt feelings by inquiring about the ingredients used or how long the dish has been sitting out. Any food brought to a public outing should be properly cooked and handled. If you are bringing food from more than two hours away, make sure it is food you can keep refrigerated and that it's eaten no longer than two hours after you make it available. Since it is difficult to regulate the temperature of hand-held coolers, make certain that all food inside the cooler is covered in ice. Don't be stingy with the ice. If you are traveling far, you may need to replenish the ice from time to time to maintain a solid layer inside the cooler at all times. Refrigerate cooked things immediately after cooking in reasonably thin, small portions so reheating the food to 165 degrees Fahrenheit will be easier when you arrive. I know it is a bother, but the friends and family who eat your casserole will appreciate that you care so much about them.

Leave cold food refrigerated until just before serving and keep it cold if you can. Do not forget that the cold food brought out on the table will fairly soon reach room temperature—especially when folks begin to dig into it. So the two-hour-at-room-temperature rule applies to cold food, too.

In Summary

- It is not wise to eat raw or rare ground meat of any kind.
- Leftovers from restaurants and the like (doggie bags) should not be eaten if the food has been at room temperature for more than two hours.
- Always remember the temperature danger zone between 40 and 140 degrees Fahrenheit.
- To be very safe, any hot leftover food stored in the refrigerator should be reheated to 165 degrees Fahrenheit before eating. If the food was a cold

item, simply do not allow the food to reach and remain at room temperature for more than two hours before the food is eaten.

- Refrigerate cooked things immediately after cooking in reasonably thin, small portions which makes reheating the food to 165 degrees Fahrenheit easier.
- Servers who prepare the food at a deli should wear protective gloves and not handle money exchanges.

Chapter Fourteen

Day Care—A Germ's Playground

The number of children in day care increased 526 percent between 1977 and 1993. This increased day-care population has led to both bad and good news. Bad news: The larger numbers of children in child-care facilities has caused 4 million to 7 million more infections each year, with an average additional cost of $30 per family to treat these infections. Good news: In a study of 1,000 children published in *The New England Journal of Medicine,* researchers have found that early childhood infections may keep children from later developing asthma.

But even with this information, you still want to protect your child from disease. So in this chapter we'll identify germ-ridden areas of day care that pose a threat to a child's health.

Are infants and toddlers more susceptible to infectious diseases?

Yes, infants and toddlers are more susceptible to germs, both bacterial and viral. There are several different reasons for this susceptibility, including the loss of Mom's passively transferred antibodies over time. During pregnancy, some of the mother's antibodies against infectious organisms or harmful substances are passed through the placenta to the fetus. After birth, if the baby is breast-fed, additional antibodies from Mom are passed to the child by this route. Together, these antibodies are the baby's protectors from the infections Mom has experienced and is experiencing in her daily life. As a result, the baby receives passive protection for at least several months against many of the potentially harmful organisms the mother may have encountered. However, when the baby is about three months of age, Mom's antibodies are almost gone from the child's bloodstream, leaving the baby at risk. And the immune response of the infant at this age and until about two years old is not fully developed.

There are other reasons for susceptibility to infection. Anyone who has watched young children knows that little kids have habits that increase their exposure to bacteria and viruses, not to mention the spread of them— they often put their fingers and pretty much anything else they can grasp into their mouths. This behavior, while normal developmentally, allows germs to enter the child's body, potentially causing an infection. Since infants and toddlers have not yet been exposed to many of the most common infectious germs, they have not yet built up their own resistance or immunity against them. For this reason many childhood immunizations begin at around two months of age—to stimulate as soon as possible the child's own immune response. A standard immunization chart for children is included later in this chapter.

What can I do to select a good child-care facility?

Every parent wants a place that is safe, a place where the caretakers are clearly concerned about the welfare of the children. You will need to do some homework to find the facility that best suits you and your child, but the work put into this initial investigation will be very much worth the effort.

A parent's best bet is to find a licensed facility to ensure that there is monitored quality control. You may contact various state and local agencies or the many resources available over the Internet for such information. If the facility is licensed, it will be inspected on a regular basis. Also, to be awarded and to maintain licensure, facilities must follow regulations that range from monitoring the minimum age of workers to checking the vaccination status of employees. These kinds of requirements help to protect children and insure a safe and healthy environment for them.

Will my child be exposed to more diseases in a child-care facility?

Yes, there is a greater likelihood for exposure to disease, but not necessarily because the day-care facility is poorly managed. We all know that children, especially toddlers, enjoy touching and placing toys or objects other than food inside their mouths. But more often than not, a child will drop the toy when it becomes obvious that it is not a cookie, and then a different child will grab it and place it in his or her mouth. No matter how well run the day-care center may be, these kinds of

Resources to help identify quality child care in your area:

- Child Care Aware: 800-424-2246
- National Resource Center for Health and Safety in Child Care: 800-598-KIDS (5437)
- The Administration for Children and Families (ACF): 202-401-9215

One great Internet location for information on child care, including licensure, is the Centers for Disease Control and Prevention's Maternal and Child Health Bureau, Health Resources and Services Administration at www.mchb.hrsa.gov. Other Web sites you can visit to obtain information on child care include:

- The ABC's of Safe and Healthy Child Care, by the CDC at www.cdc.gov/ncidod/hip/abc/contents.htm
- NCCIC—National Child Care Information Center at ericps.crc.uiuc.edu/nccic/statepro.html
- U.S. Department of Health and Human Services, the Administration for Children and Families at www.acf.dhhs.gov

interactions are, for the most part, inevitable—especially if there are babies and very young children present. However, there are data from the CDC and other sources that show that well-run day-care facilities are not necessarily any worse as *sources* of disease outbreaks than other places in the community. In fact, the level of illness within day-care centers tends to reflect what's going around in the community. But, like any place where many people gather and interact closely, a day-care center can increase the chance of transmission of illnesses among the staff and kids. The daily

> **Information from the FDA:** Statistics have shown that cases of diarrheal illnesses are at least 30 percent more common in children in day care as opposed to children cared for at home.

interaction can lead to rapid transfer of illness among the children and, subsequently, among the caretakers and parents, causing repeating cycles of illness to occur.

What are the most common illnesses in day-care centers?

Other than the common cold, the most common illnesses among children in day care are those associated with an upset stomach and/or diarrhea. Different bacteria and viruses that can cause these problems, several of which you will recognize from previous chapters, including such viruses as hepatitis A and rotavirus, bacteria such as *Campylobacter,* and parasites such as *Cryptosporidium.* While these germs may be transmitted to the children and workers in water or food, these sources are not usually an issue in well-managed day-care centers. Rather, fecal contamination due to the caring for the child in diapers or fecal contamination of the caretaker's hands or the child's hands after bowel movements are the usual source of the problem and will be discussed in depth later in this chapter. Therefore, those who see to the children must be careful to keep things clean.

Is there any way to reduce the child's risk of illness while in day care?

It is almost impossible to prevent children from digging in the dirt and sharing cookies, both of which increase the amount of germs to which they are exposed. Along with the close environment, the presence of very small children still in diapers increases the possibility that some kind of bacterial or viral infection can be rapidly spread. So it is particularly important for

---

From the CDC: Immunization recommendations for child-care facility employees and workers generally include: influenza, measles, mumps and rubella (MMR), tetanus and diphtheria (Td), polio, hepatitis A, chickenpox, hepatitis B (if they encounter blood through work with developmentally disabled or aggressive children). Also, employees generally should have received a tuberculin skin test to check for the presence of tuberculosis.

---

both parents and day-care providers to know how to hamper the spread of pathogens.

Vaccinations go a long way toward preventing illness and the possibility of transmission of an infectious disease. Unless the germs gain a foothold and increase in number, they cannot be spread. Vaccinations prevent either the foothold from ever being gained or the growth of the germ in question. Consequently, be sure to ask to see the facility's immunization record for each employee. Given the personal nature of the question, it may be difficult to ask, but the availability of these records is an important indicator of the risk your child may face. If this record is not available or if the facility refuses to release the information, I might look for another facility.

If the child-care setting is a home and people other than employees live there, ask to see their immunization records too. You should also expect the facility to ask for your child's immunization record. If they do not ask you, again, consider taking your child somewhere else. Be familiar with which immunizations the Centers for Disease Control recommends for child-care personnel.

What are some of the things a day-care center can do to prevent infections?

While we seem to keep coming back to the procedure of hand-washing no matter what the topic, an estimated 50 percent of intestinally related illnesses could be prevented by this simple act. A special antibacterial kind of soap is not required: Regular soap is fine since the goal of the hand washing is the removal of all types of germs from the surfaces and crevices.

Recommended Childhood Immunization Schedule
United States, January–December 2000

Vaccine	Age (in order of best age to receive vaccinations)
Hepatitis B	Birth to 2 months 1–4 months *11–12 years
Diphtheria, Tetanus, Pertussis	15–18 months 2–6 months
H. Influenzae Type B	12–15 months 2–6 months
Polio	6–18 months 2–6 months
Measles, mumps, rubella	12–15 months 2–6 months *4–6 years
Varicella	12–18 months *11–12 years
Hepatitis A	24 months–12 years

*Indicates ages vaccinations may be given if previously recommended dosages were missed or given earlier than recommended age.

Day Care—A Germ's Playground

1. This schedule indicates the recommended ages for routine administration of currently licensed childhood vaccines as of 11/1/99. Additional vaccines may be licensed and recommended during the year. Licensed combination vaccines may be used whenever any components of the combination are indicated and its other components are not contraindicated. Providers should consult manufacturers' package inserts for detailed recommendations.

2. *Infants born to HBsAg-negative mothers* should receive the first dose of hepatitis B (Hep B) vaccine by age 2 months. The second dose should be at least 1 month after the first dose. The third dose should be administered at least 4 months after the first dose and at least 2 months after the second dose, but not before 6 months of age for infants.

Infants born to HBsAg-positive mothers should receive hepatitis B vaccine and 0.5 mL hepatitis B immune globulin (HBIG) within 12 hours of birth at separate sites. The second dose is recommended at 1 to 2 months of age, and the third dose at 6 months of age.

Infants born to mothers whose HBsAg status is unknown should receive hepatitis B vaccine within 12 hours of birth. Maternal blood should be drawn at the time of delivery to determine the mother's HBsAg status; if the HBsAg test is positive, the infant should receive HBIG as soon as possible (no later than 1 week of age).

Children and adolescents (through 18 years of age) who have not been immunized against hepatitis B may begin the series during any visit. Special care should be taken as to children who were born in or whose parents were born in areas of the world with moderate or high endemicity of hepatitis B virus infection.

3. The fourth dose of DTaP (diphtheria and tetanus toxoids and acellular pertussis vaccine) may be administered as early as 12 months of age, provided 6 months have elapsed since the third dose and the child is unlikely to return at age 15 to 18 months. Td (tetanus and diphtheria toxoids) is recommended at 11 to 12 years of age if at least 5 years have elapsed since the last dose of DTP, DTaP, or DT. Subsequent routine Td boosters are recommended every 10 years.

4. Three *Haemophilus influenzae* Type B (Hib) conjugate vaccines are licensed for infant use. If PRP-OMP is administered at 2

211

and 4 months of age, a dose at 6 months is not required. Because clinical studies in infants have demonstrated that using some combination products may induce a lower immune response to the Hib vaccine component, DTaP/Hib combination products should not be used for primary immunization in infants at 2, 4, or 6 months of age, unless FDA-approved for these ages.

5. To eliminate the risk of vaccine-associated paralytic polio (VAPP), an all-IPV (inactivated polio vaccine) schedule is now recommended for routine childhood polio vaccination in the United States.

All children should receive four doses of IPV at 2 months, 4 months, 6 to 18 months, and 4 to 6 years. Oral polio vaccine (live, attenuated), (OPV), if available, may be used only for the following special circumstances:

1. Mass vaccination campaigns to control outbreaks of paralytic polio.
2. Unvaccinated children who will be traveling in less than 4 weeks to areas where polio is endemic or epidemic.
3. Children of parents who do not accept the recommended number of vaccine injections. These children may receive OPV only for the third or fourth dose or both; in this situation, health-care providers should administer OPV only after discussing the risk for VAPP with parents or caregivers.
4. During the transition to an all-IPV schedule, recommendations for the use of remaining OPV supplies in physicians' offices and clinics have been issued by the American Academy of Pediatrics (see *Pediatrics,* December 1999).

6. The second dose of measles, mumps, and rubella (MMR) vaccine is recommended routinely at 4 to 6 years of age but may be administered during any visit, provided at least 4 weeks have elapsed since receipt of the first dose and that both doses are administered beginning at or after 12 months of age. Those who have not previously received the second dose should complete the schedule by the 11 or 12-year-old visit.

7. Varicella (Var) vaccine is recommended at any visit on or

after the first birthday for susceptible children, i.e., those who lack a reliable history of chickenpox (as judged by a health-care provider) and who have not been immunized. Susceptible persons 13 years of age or older should receive 2 doses, given at least 4 weeks apart.

8. Hepatitis A (Hep A) for recommended use in selected states and/or regions; consult your local public health authority.

All kids should wash their hands or have their hands washed upon arrival at day-care. Everyone's hands at the center should again be washed before preparing food and before eating anything, as well as after any trip to the bathroom or after changing a child's diaper. Check on this policy at your day-care center from time to time, and be sure that it is carried out.

Another area that is worth mentioning, as small as it seems, is the length of the staff's fingernails. *Pseudomonas aeruginosa* is a bacterium that can live in fairly high concentration underneath long fingernails—this same bug, you might remember, can contaminate eye make-up and can cause severe eye infections. In fact, it was recently reported that a hospital intensive care unit determined that deaths of neonatal intensive care infants were due to exposure to this bacterium, which was subsequently found underneath the long fingernails of nursing staff. While it is impossible to determine whether or not the nurses had transmitted the bacterium to these infants, there is enough concern to warrent awareness of this potential problem. Therefore, it is probably best if the staff has short fingernails. Alternatively, any person with long nails should take extra special care to clean underneath them, while keeping in mind that the usual hand-washing procedures may not be enough.

Food preparation is also a concern at day-care centers, particularly if there are a number of meals served. Good kitchen hygiene should be expected, but ask how food is prepared and how leftovers are handled. The same risks of food-borne illness that we have already discussed in the kitchen and food chapters apply here as well. If there are infants and toddlers who are receiving milk in the form of formula, it is imperative that the bottles are boiled before use.

If mothers provide breast milk, it should be fresh and either refrigerated or frozen for later use. Breast milk, which is naturally sterile, contains cells and proteins that are antibacterial and is therefore better in this regard for the child than formula. So if the milk is collected in a sterile container, the chances of the child getting one of the intestinal bugs are lessened.

What should I do if my child is ill or if the other kids become ill?

Day-care facilities should provide parents with written information that fully describes the policy on handling children who are ill. Normally, any child with diarrhea or a cold, flu, or any other kind of respiratory illness should not be placed in close contact with the other children. Germs that cause these illnesses are easily transferred from person to person, even under the best of conditions. By the same token, a child should not be taken to the facility for care if he or she is ill and might be contagious. It is simply not fair to the other children or their parents.

Centers may have varying policies on what to do when a child has a fever. For example, the American Academy of Pediatrics recommends that a child with a fever not be taken to child care. On the other hand, the National Health and Safety Performance Standards (NHSPS) established by the National Resource Center for Health and Safety in Child Care recommend that a child with a fever be kept at home only if additional complications or symptoms of illness are present (such as coughing, diarrhea, or rash). In this situation, choose the policy you prefer. In any case, depending on the facility, if your child becomes ill, you should expect to be contacted. Make sure that such a procedure exists.

How should the center clean toys?

Toys can bring different risks of bug transmission, and there should be a routine procedure for cleaning them. Plastic or hard-surfaced toys are easier to clean than soft-surfaced ones, but all toys should be washed. Hard-surfaced toys should be washed at the end of every day, or at least before the next day's onslaught of little ones. Any soft toys with smooth fabric or a furry exterior should be run through a washing machine with water hotter than 140 degrees Fahrenheit once a week.

What about cleaning other things besides toys?

Toys are not the only items that need routine cleaning. The day-care facility should make sure that any surfaces a child may touch with hands or mouth, like benches, slides, and the crib rails, are routinely cleaned. Areas where food is prepared should be thoroughly and routinely cleaned as well. There should be a separate sink or sinks for food preparation.

Good old soap and water and elbow grease will usually get the job done in most areas. However, the diaper area and bathrooms should have a stronger treatment, preferably a disinfectant. A higher-strength diluted bleach solution is effective. The CDC recommends 1/4 cup of bleach (5.25 percent sodium hypochlorite) added to one gallon of cool water (or one tablespoon of bleach added to one quart of cool water) for disinfecting bathrooms and diapering areas.

If diluted bleach is not used, just be sure that the center uses a product that meets the Environmental Protection Agency's standards for hospital-grade germicides, which will kill disease-causing viruses, bacteria, and parasites. A hospital-grade disinfectant (germicide) must bear an EPA registration number. This number is a certification of EPA disinfectant standards and is required for all products labeled as disinfectants. Some of these products may be obtained at the local supermarket, and as long as there is an EPA registration number, any product will behave similarly. However, stronger disinfectants may not normally be available. In this instance, if such stringent disinfecting is called for, a physician or pharmacist will need to be contacted in order to locate a source.

If a child becomes ill and has played with toys or touched surfaces, workers should disinfect these items rather than depend only upon soap-and-water cleaning.

What other precautions can the day-care center take?

There are several additional precautions the people running the day-care center can enact to prevent the spread of infection among the children. There should be a separate place for changing diapers and its surface should not be covered, meaning that no absorbent material should be underneath the child unless it is disposable. Also, the container for disposable diapers should not be accessible to the rest of the kids.

After a diaper is changed, the area should be disinfected with either a commercial disinfectant that can kill bacteria, viruses, and parasites (a hospital-grade disinfectant) or with the bleach solution we have discussed (one tablespoon of bleach in one quart of water). The bleach must be allowed to remain on the area for several minutes—a quick swipe will not suffice. Then the surfaces should be rinsed well because bleach can be caustic to the skin, especially a child's. If a bleach solution is used, the solution should be prepared daily and stored away from direct sunlight, as it loses effectiveness over time. A cautionary note: *Never* mix bleach with anything but water or soap. Mixing bleach with other chemicals (especially ammonia) can sometimes lead to the production of chlorine gas, which is highly toxic.

Young children, especially those still in diapers, should have their own place to play apart from the older kids. Also, any child who has a bout of diarrhea while at the day-care center should be separated from the other children. While a child is recovering from an intestinal illness of some kind, the child may still be a carrier of the organism and will shed the organism in the stool over several days, even after the diarrhea completely subsides. Consequently, any child who has recovered from a case of diarrhea should be kept apart from the other kids for a day or two, just in case the child is still carrying something that could be transmitted. If the day-care center follows these relatively straightforward practices, the chance of spreading contagious diseases is greatly reduced.

Are there risks to be found in toothbrushes and hairbrushes?

The day-care facility (and you) should make certain that all toothbrushes are kept separate from one another and that children do not share them. Ask the staff if there are new toothbrushes available just in case the kids decide to trade brushes with each other. Lots of diseases can be transmitted via the bacteria and viruses on the brush hairs, including, for example, *Streptococcus pyogenes,* the bacterium that causes strep throat.

Similarly, children should have their own hairbrush and no brush should ever be shared among the rest of the kids. Not only bacteria but also fungi and head lice can be spread among the children if hairbrushes are shared.

In Summary

- Until about age two, infants and toddlers are more susceptible to bacterial and viral infections.
- Other than the common cold, the most common

illnesses among children in day care are those associated with an upset stomach and/or diarrhea.

There are several different bacteria and viruses that can cause these problems, including such viruses as hepatitis A, enteric adenovirus, and rotavirus, and bacteria such as *Campylobacter,* and parasites such as *Cryptosporidium.*

- As much as a 50 percent reduction in intestinally related illnesses could be prevented by the simple act of hand-washing. Consequently, all kids should wash their hands or have their hands washed upon arrival at day care.
- Hard-surfaced toys should be washed at the end of every day, or at least before the next day's onslaught of little ones. Any soft toys with smooth fabric or a furry exterior should be run through a washing machine with water hotter than 140 degrees Fahrenheit once a week.
- Young children, especially those in diapers, should have their own place to play apart from the older kids.
- Children should never share a toothbrush or a hairbrush with anyone.
- Day-care facilities should provide parents with written information that fully describes the policy on handling children who are ill.

Chapter Fifteen

How Healthy Is
Your Health-Care Facility?

Considering the care that goes into keeping a hospital sanitary, a surprising number of infections can result from a stay in a hospital or other health-care facility.

What is the risk of getting an infection in these situations?

Any infection acquired while in a hospital or other health-care facility is known as a nosocomial infection (the word *nosocomial* is derived from the Greek; *nosos,* "disease," and *komeion,* "to take care of"). There is a strange irony that we can enter a hospital without an infection and get one while we are there. Unfortunately, an estimated 2 million to 2 1/2 million of these infections occur annually in the United States, and the rate of such infections has increased 36 percent in the last twenty years. They can pose significant health risks to the patient. Nosocomial infections lead directly or contribute to approximately 100,000 deaths each year in the United States. These infections are expensive to treat, as well, estimated to exceed $4 1/2 billion annually.

Equally disturbing is that nosocomial infections represent over 50 percent of all of the complications suffered during hospitalization.

How is it possible to acquire an infection while in a hospital?

Obviously, there are sick people inside a hospital. And whenever anyone enters a hospital, he or she may bring infectious microbes along. Anytime the protective layer of our skin is broken, such as with surgery, our risk of infection is increased. Depending on the extent of the surgery or the state of our health at the time, our ability to fight off the bug is compromised. Too, certain conditions like cancer or HIV infection increase the risk of a bacterial infection. Unfortunately, no matter how careful a hospital may be, there is just no way to eradicate infectious organisms completely. Remember, they are on our skin, inside our mouths and noses—everywhere.

Further, if for whatever reason our intestinal flora are not in proper proportions, such as after extensive surgery or trauma, it is possible for intestinal organisms to transfer into our bloodstream and tissues (the medical term for this is bacterial translocation). When we are physically traumatized, there appears to be a breakdown in our normal protective systems. If a pathogen is present in the intestines, even in low numbers, under such circumstances the bug can cross over into adjacent tissues and perhaps into the bloodstream. Additionally, since doctors, nurses, and other staff must touch us in order to help us, they can transfer germs to us, thus placing us at higher risk for an infection.

221

When are we more likely to get an infection?

As the cost of health care has increased dramatically, the length of stays in health-care facilities, particularly in hospitals, has shortened. As a consequence, outpatient care has become more common. This trend has resulted in making hospitals places of extended care for only the very seriously ill. This change means that the majority of patients who remain in the hospital are, because of the serious nature of their conditions, much more vulnerable to any infection they might get.

Who is particularly at risk?

Burn, surgical and trauma patients, the elderly no matter their initial condition, and anyone whose immune system is not functioning well are particularly at risk.

If a person is burned, the immune system can be severely compromised as a result. One of our body's responses to the trauma of a burn is to produce substances that severely block the ability of the immune system to function properly. Nobody knows why our bodies respond in this way—you'd think it would be just the opposite—but they do. A burn also leads to the loss of the outer protective layer of skin, and if the burn is second or third degree, the damage can be to deeper tissues as well. This non-protected, exposed tissue allows germs a rich place to attach and to grow. A common risk that burn patients must deal with is an infection caused by *Pseudomonas aeruginosa,* which on its own accounts for approximately 8 percent of all nosocomial infections. This organism can grow extensively in the tissues and can result in an overwhelming infection and the death of the patient. That is why burn patients are isolated in a special burn unit where very stringent procedures are constantly followed.

A similar thing happens to the immune system if a person is severely injured or has undergone major surgery (abdominal surgery, for example). The body's response to injury has an adverse effect on a number of different physiologic systems, and one of them is the immune system. Thus, any infectious agent will have a better opportunity to establish itself and cause serious problems. As a consequence, there are a number of special units for each surgical procedure or other condition. These units are: neonatal (NICU), pediatric (PICU), surgical (SICU), medical (MICU)—for all non-surgical patients, such as those with pneumonia—cardiac (CICU), and, in some hospitals, maternal-fetal (MFICU) and burn (BICU).

What are the risks of surgery?

Surgery exposes the body to the potential for infection, but precautions are taken to keep the patient safe from any stray germs. All of the equipment and all of the implements used in the operating room are sterile. The staff involved are also covered from head to toe with sterile clothing and are disinfected to reduce the possibility of transferring a germ to the patient. Surgeons vigorously scrub their hands and arms with disinfectant for ten to fifteen minutes to remove the outer layer of dead skin (where germs can be hiding out) and to kill any bugs that remain.

The patient's body is also disinfected, though not as extensively. The skin and gown of the patient are cleaned, but not necessarily sterilized, and the area of the body exposed to surgery will be disinfected with a powerful anti-germ solution. This procedure generally prevents a bug that might be on the body from reaching the wound. If the goal of the surgery is to remove an ongoing infection such as an abscess of some sort, a germ may be released from the abscess into the patient's

---

Data from the CDC reveal that nosocomial infections are caused by the following microorganisms (percentages are rounded up):

- 34 percent are due to three gram-positive organisms—*Staphylococcus aureus, Enterococcus* species, and other species of *Staphylococcus.*
- 32 percent are due to four different gram-negative bacteria—*Klebsiella pneumoniae, Escherichia coli, Enterobacter* species, and *Pseudomonas aeruginosa.*
- 18 percent are respiratory infections caused by *S. aureus, Enterobacter* species, and *Pseudomonas aeruginosa.*
- 17 percent are site infections caused by *S. aureus* and *Enterococcus.*

Left untreated, any one of these infections can lead to death by pneumonia or sepsis.

---

surrounding tissue or into the bloodstream. In these instances, the person will receive extensive antibiotic therapy as a precaution to prevent the possibility of infection.

Also, certain kinds of surgery may require that a tube be introduced into the patient to perform functions such as draining fluid, providing nutrients, or assisting breathing. Tubes offer a particularly good place for germs to enter unprotected areas of the body through a direct route. Health-care personnel are fully aware of this risk and take steps to prevent infection. Patients with tubes are periodically tested at the point of entry of such tubes and IVs, and any bacteria present are cultured for identification in the bacteriological laboratory of the hospital. If there is evidence of bacterial growth, appropriate antibiotic therapy is given right away.

What are supergerms?

The abundant use of antibiotics in health-care facilities creates an environment that enables resistant germs to be selected and therefore to become dominant (all others are sensitive and, therefore, are killed). These germs have mutated or have somehow otherwise acquired the ability to become resistant to a given antibiotic. In a relatively closed ecological place like a health-care facility, the organisms that reside there are under fairly constant environmental stresses. If the common presence of antibiotics is one of the stressors, those bugs that are sensitive will be killed. Those bugs that aren't killed develop a sort of mechanism to resist the effect of the antibiotic, allowing them to survive and thrive. Antibiotic-resistant strains of *Staphylococcus aureus* and certain strains of *Enterococcus* species are particularly worrisome. Some members of these groups have become resistant to methicillin, an antibiotic that is a derivative of penicillin that's often used to treat such infections.

Vancomycin is often considered by the public to be the antibiotic "of last resort," and its use is commonly thought to be limited to the most severe cases of infection. However, because of legitimate concern about antibiotic-resistant bacteria, the use of vancomycin has dramatically increased as a preventative tool to fight infections, particularly in surgical intensive-care units. As a consequence, bacteria resistant to vancomycin have now emerged. These antibiotic-resistant strains are not more infectious, nor are they necessarily more harmful in their action. Health-care professionals are concerned, however, that if an infection occurs from these particular bugs, treatment will become more difficult.

As a patient, what can I do about this situation?

Assertiveness when being treated can prevent contracting an infection. Ask the doctor or nurse please to wash his or her hands before examining you. This single act may be the very thing that prevents you from acquiring an infection. Several studies show that, depending on the facility examined, approximately 14 to 59 percent of doctors and from 25 to 45 percent of nurses regularly wash their hands between patients. According to these estimates, doctors and nurses could reduce nosocomial infections by at least 50 percent through the simple act of washing their hands between patient examinations. In fact, studies have shown that only about 10 percent of patients will ask doctors or nurses to wash their hands or ask them if they have before the examination, even if there is a program in the hospital that encourages this policy.

Another thing you can do is to inquire about the occurrence of such infections inside the facility. There will usually be a person on staff, known as the infection control nurse or epidemiologist, who is responsible for tracking infections throughout the hospital and who will be able to answer any questions you may have. So be as proactive as you can. Certainly, if you are too ill to investigate this issue, ask a friend or relative to take on this rather uncomfortable task. Similarly, if you have a relative or a friend who is unable to ask or is too embarrassed to ask about hand-washing procedures, you might consider doing an important favor by asking on his or her behalf.

Why can't children visit hospitals?

The reason children are often barred from hospitals is because their presence increases the potential for spread of infectious bugs—either from the child to the patient or vice versa. In general, small kids are rambunctious and you would certainly not want a toddler to wander accidentally into a rack holding intravenous fluids. If you think about it, the hospital is just not the best place for children—there is too much risk of infection in both directions, and too much risk of injury to the child and to the patient. So it is best to have little ones stay at home.

227

Are nursing homes safe?

The risk that a resident of a nursing home will acquire an infection is significant too. People in nursing homes are usually elderly (in 1997 the average age for female residents was eighty-three, and the average age for male residents was seventy-six) and are often in relatively poor health. Their immune function is not quite as good in comparison to that of young adults. The weakened immune system makes them significantly more vulnerable to infection, particularly the respiratory kind. That is why it is so strongly recommended that these individuals as well as the staff caring for them receive immunization against the influenza viruses. Also, anyone aged sixty-five or older should be immunized with the pneumococcal (pneumococcal polysaccharide) vaccine to protect them from bacterial pneumonia.

However, nosocomial infections can also readily be acquired, particularly *Staphylococcus, Enterococcus,* or *E. coli.* Another concern is antibiotic-resistant bugs in this environment. So, just as in the hospital, the staff should be asked to wash their hands before caring for one of these elderly patients. If you have a loved one who is staying in a nursing home, you might want to check around to see the availability of strong anti-germ cleaning agents. These agents often contain something called chlorhexidine, which is a very good hospital-grade antibacterial and antiviral disinfecting agent. Ask the staff occasionally if there are any antibiotic-resistant cases in the facility and, if so, what precautions are being taken to protect other residents.

Pay attention to general procedures and how clean

the facility appears, and be aware of any bad odors. Make sure you do not visit when you are ill, particularly if you have cold or flu symptoms. Be sure to wash your hands thoroughly before visiting and after you leave. Just try to keep in mind that these folks are a bit more physically frail and you may need to take some extra precautions to protect them from any harmful germs.

In Summary

- Whenever we are admitted as a patient in a hospital, we are at higher risk for acquiring an infection while there.
- Infections acquired while within a health-care facility are known as nosocomial infections.
- The number of nosocomial infections is increasing, but not necessarily because hospitals aren't doing a decent job. Since the average hospital stay has decreased, the percentage of patients who remain in hospital are significantly more ill than in the past and are therefore at higher risk for infection.
- Burn wounds, surgery, physical trauma, cancer, and other diseases make us more vulnerable to infection.
- Antibiotic-resistant organisms are on the increase, particularly in health-care facilities. Two of the major culprits are methicillin-resistant *Staphylococcus aureus* (MRSA) and vancomycin-resistant *Enterococcus* (VRE).
- Young children should not visit a hospital patient

unless specifically allowed to do so by the patient's physician.

- If you are a patient, respectfully ask the doctor and nurse if they have washed their hands prior to examining you.
- Nursing-home residents are at risk for nosocomial infections too. And because of the relatively older age of these residents, they are particularly vulnerable to respiratory infections.
- Anyone aged sixty-five or older should be immunized with the pneumococcal (pneumococcal polysaccharide) vaccine to protect them from bacterial pneumonia.

Chapter Sixteen

The Wide World of Germs–
Travel and Vacations

Most people enjoy seeing new places and doing new things, but wherever you roam, those pesky germs are sure to follow. In your travels, you may even run into some new ones that are unfamiliar. In this chapter we will focus on some of the more common bugs and potential health problems you may face while away from home.

Is there an increased chance that I will catch something while I am traveling?

Staying in any confined space with other people for an extended period of time increases the risk of catching an infectious bug. Regardless of whether you are on a plane, train, bus, or tooling around on the open sea in a cruise ship, if you are with other people, you will come in contact with their germs. Basic sanitation practices, such as hand-washing and avoiding touching your eyes, nose, and mouth, are doubly important in these circumstances. But if you are traveling in an underdeveloped country, the risk increases because sanitation conditions are not as dependable as they are in developed countries.

231

According to the Centers for Disease Control, between 15 to 50 percent of all travelers to developing countries contract some illness during or after travel, with about 5 percent of these needing medical attention. The most common infections in returned travelers involve gastrointestinal infections with diarrhea, which affects from 20 to 40 percent of short-term travelers. The most common life-threatening infections are malaria, viral hepatitis, and amoebiasis.

Washing your hands with contaminated water will not help stop the spread of disease.

The lack of consistent cleanliness is why immunizations are required. While we cannot do much to avoid colds, we can avoid coming down with the flu or other illnesses simply by becoming immunized against prevalent diseases. When staying in a country with less-than-perfect sanitation conditions, be aware that you may not have protection against the same germs as the natives. The World Health Organization's Web site (www.who.int) lists current outbreaks of particular diseases occurring around the world. This gives you a good opportunity to see what diseases you may run into and allows you to be able to take some additional precautions.

Are immunizations important only for foreign travel or for domestic travel as well?

No matter where you plan to travel or what you plan to do, one of the best things you can do to prepare for your trip is to update your immunizations. In general, traveling in a developed, industrialized country is not any riskier from a germ standpoint than traveling within the United States. Therefore, the standard list of recommended vaccinations is usually sufficient protection when you are in any developed nation. Some of these will depend on the particular country you plan to visit and may even be required by that nation before you are allowed to visit. Many of these special vaccinations will depend upon whether you are staying in a town or a city, or in the rural areas of the countryside. And finally, depending on the area and how you plan to spend your time there, especially if you are camping or hiking, there may be even more specific vaccine recommendations.

Recommendations are made by the Advisory Committee on Immunization Practices (ACIP) of the United States with material published at the Centers for Disease Control and Prevention (CDC). With the enormous amount of useful information about immunizations provided by the CDC's Web site (www.cdc.gov), the specific site, http://wonder.cdc.gov/wonder/prev-guid/m0025228/entire.htm, details all of the different immunizations needed for travel both inside and outside the United States, as well as links to individual countries.

Are planes on par with petri dishes?

Outside an airborne jet the air is unbreathable. Therefore, air packs are used to pressurize the outside air, which is then combined with recycled air and circulated within the jet's cabin. However, according to

For people traveling within the United States, ACIP recommends:

- Vaccinations against measles, mumps, rubella, polio, tetanus, diphtheria, and pertussis, and, for those over sixty-five years of age, pneumococcal polysaccharide.
- As of April 2000 it is recommended that persons fifty years of age and older receive influenza vaccination.
- For children, vaccination against measles, mumps, rubella, polio, tetanus, diphtheria, pertussis, *Haemophilus influenzae* Type B (conjugate vaccine), and hepatitis B are recommended.

For travelers outside the United States, recommended immunizations include:

- Those against hepatitis B, rabies, meningococcal polysaccharide, yellow fever, typhoid, cholera, and plague—depending upon the area to be visited and sometimes the potential for unavoidable contact with wild animals.
- For malaria, the recommended treatment is a chemical preventative, to be taken before travel, while at your destination, and for a time after you return. Contact your physician if you plan to travel to an area where malaria is prevalent. You will likely be prescribed either mefloquine or doxycycline.

the airplane manufacturers, planes that recirculate air have HEPA (high-efficiency particulate-arresting) filters in their air-handling systems. HEPA filters, which are recommended by the CDC for use in hospitals to protect persons from diseases such as tuberculosis, are able to filter out most bacteria from the air.

There is not a lot you can do to avoid germs on a plane except get a flu vaccination every fall and ask to be moved if you are seated next to someone who appears to be sick. And don't rush to preboard: Ventilation is worse before takeoff and after landing.

Is there any harm to be found on a sea cruise?

Cruise ships can be like little floating cities. Consequently, the same germy problems you might encounter in any city may be encountered here as well. Cruise ships need to be particularly careful of disease outbreak because illness can spread rapidly in the confined parameters of the ship, and among the members of the crew as well as the passengers.

A ship at sea must produce all of its own water, using large distillation units aboard to convert seawater to freshwater. If your ship's engine is steam-driven, most of the precious water will be used to power the ship in one form or the other. The rest, however, known as potable water, will be stored for human use. All of the water used for showering, bathing, and drinking must be properly and continuously treated in order to kill germs and prevent contamination of the ship's storage tanks and water-supply lines.

Additionally, a ship must carry all of its food and

supplies while at sea, and unless there are frequent port stops, there may not be frequent replenishment of these items. As a consequence, longer storage periods may be the norm. While aboard, you should also keep in mind the dangers associated with food handling and preparation, the same concerns outlined in Chapters Nine and Thirteen.

The CDC reports that every vessel that has a foreign itinerary, carries thirteen or more passengers, and calls on a U.S. port is subject to unannounced twice-yearly inspections and, when necessary, to re-inspection by Vessel Sanitation Program staff. The vessel owner pays a fee, based on tonnage, for all inspections. Currently, more than 140 cruise ships participate in the program.

The inspections are conducted by environmental health officers (EHOs) of the Vessel Sanitation Program, and take place only in U.S. ports. The inspection may take from five to eight hours to complete, depending on the size and complexity of the vessel. The ships must meet the criteria established by VSP in the *Vessel Sanitation Program Operations Manual*. The ship is given a score based on a 100-point scale. To pass the inspection, a ship must score 86 or above. If the ship fails an inspection, it will be reinspected, usually within thirty to forty-five days.

Is there any truth to the common "Do Not Drink the Water" advice?

In underdeveloped nations where sanitation conditions are substandard, water is often contaminated. Eating uncooked food or food washed with tap water, such as fruits or vegetables, can be a risky venture. In some cases it is recommended that you do all of your food preparation yourself. But keep in mind that the water you use for washing or cooking food may be contaminated. For example, seventy tourists from the United Kingdom who drank only bottled water while staying in a hotel in Greece were still stricken with the water-borne pathogen *Giardia lamblia,* a germ that causes gastrointestinal illness. Their illness could have been caused by something as simple as brushing their teeth with tap water. Therefore, depending on where you are, you should boil any water you use for food preparation and certainly before drinking.

Because of the significantly increased risk of such ill-

From the CDC: "In areas with poor sanitation, only the following beverages may be safe to drink: boiled water, hot beverages made with boiled water such as coffee or tea, canned or bottled carbonated beverages, beer, and wine. Ice may be made from unsafe water and should be avoided. It is safer to drink a beverage from a can or bottle than to drink from a container that was not known to be clean and dry. However, water on the surface of a beverage can or bottle may also be contaminated. Therefore, the area of a can or bottle that will touch the mouth should be wiped clean and dry. In areas where water is contaminated, travelers should not brush their teeth with tap water."

nesses in underdeveloped countries, find out the conditions of the place before you visit. If you are eating out in any of these countries, consider not eating any uncooked food and not drinking anything that has not been significantly heated or does not appear in a can or bottle. Do not forget about the ice—just because the water has been frozen does not mean it will not make you ill.

How clean is the average hotel room?

Travelers often assume that hotel personnel are just as conscientious as they are about making a room clean and germ-free. Unfortunately, this is not always the case, as an article concerning hotel cleanliness on www.globalassignment.com reports. Hotel staff often cut corners when cleaning the rooms; management sometimes instructs their employees to spend less than ten minutes on each room in between check-out and check-in time during a busy season, making it impossible for the employees to do much more than straighten up.

For example, instead of completely replacing the used bed linens, one former hotel employee states that some hotel cleaning services may simply remake the bed with the old sheets and covers, smoothing out the top bedspread or sheet so that there appears to be a fresh set of linens on the bed. Another area a housekeeping service is often tempted to skimp on is the bathroom and shower. Sinks, counters, and bathtubs (which are supposed to be thoroughly sanitized with an industrial cleaner) are more often than not given a quick "wipe job," many times with the wet bath towel left behind by the previous guest. To be on the safe side, closely inspect the bedding before you decide to settle in for your stay. Do the sheets, pillowcases, and towels look and smell clean? If you have any doubt in your mind, contact the main desk and request a complete linen change. If you want to be on the safe side, apply a spray disinfectant to a cloth and wipe down all surfaces such as doorknobs, faucets, and desktops.

What germs will be there to greet me in the great outdoors?

Many people absolutely love wandering around in the wild for days on end and can settle down in a tent or sleeping bag without the slightest bit of discomfort. I love camping too—as long as, at the end of a long day, I have a comfortable bed and hot shower waiting for me at a hotel. Whether I am asking where the nearest hotel might be or you are rappelling off a cliff in Yosemite, the one thing we both want to avoid is an infection or a reaction from an insect's sting or bite.

Before you start out on your hiking or camping adventure, get as much information as you can about the availability and condition of the water in the areas you plan to visit. Unless you are planning to go pretty deep into the wilderness, information exists on the possible dangers of the water supply. If you plan to stay in a wilderness area in the United States, a member of the National Park Service or the U.S. Forestry Service in the area may be able to tell you of potential contamination dangers. If you are not in the United States it is a good idea to contact local government agencies in the area for advice. As a precaution in the wild, always assume water will be contaminated.

If deer drink out of a stream, why can't I?

If you spend the day hiking all over the woods, sooner or later you will get thirsty. As you look down into that cold, clear, sparkling stream, just keep looking, and then walk on to the nearest campground to find potable water. Always remember that if you are out in the wild, the water will likely be wild too. There can be some pretty awful germs in stream, river, or lake (surface) water, the majority of which will also thrive in our intestinal tract.

Along with various viruses and bacteria, water is often teeming with the troublesome intestinal parasite (a protozoan) known as *Giardia*. This germ is shed in the fecal matter of wild animals and will easily contaminate streams and rivers. If you happen to become infected with this bug, the infection can be treated but you will probably be miserable for quite a while. Another bad water bug, *Cryptosporidium,* is commonly found in streams and rivers, as well as in any type of surface water. This protozoan can cause significant illness and can possibly be fatal if your immune system is not working well.

Because of the fairly high possibility of swallowing some nasty germ from outdoor streams and rivers, all of the water you drink should either be packed with you from home or boiled for at least ten minutes if you obtain it from the wild. If you plan to be at higher elevations, remember that water boils at a temperature lower than 212 degrees Fahrenheit, so boil the water for a longer period of time. If you can't boil the water you get from a stream, then you can use water purification tablets that contain chlorine or iodine.

Some folks additionally recommend water filters, but others feel that these systems aren't always reliable. One thing to keep in mind when using iodine-based water purification tablets is that you shouldn't use them for too many days at a time. Extended use of these tablets may lead to problems with the thyroid. So be careful, especially if you happen to have any kind of thyroid condition that's being treated (talk with your physician and your pharmacist about your plans). Also keep in mind that both *Giardia* and *Cryptosporidium* are tough to kill with purification tablets alone because they can exist in an intermediate and very tough cyst form. This form of the bugs, along with bacteria and viruses is, thank goodness, sensitive to heat. Therefore, it is best to boil the water to get rid of any infectious microorganisms.

What about Ebola?

The *Ebola* virus causes a form of viral hemorrhagic fever and you have very little chance of contracting it while traveling (which is amazing, considering the news coverage). There are four different families of viruses that can cause viral hemorrhagic fevers: filoviruses, of which *Ebola* is a member, along with members of the arenavirus, flavivirus, and bunyavirus families. The source of the *Ebola* virus (the natural reservoir) in nature is unknown. However, because of the occurrence of these other, similar viruses in animals (rodents, for example) *Ebola* is thought to reside in an animal host as well, somewhere on the continent of Africa. Although the source of the virus in nature is unknown, it can occasionally be found in rodents, ticks, and mosquitoes within endemic areas. Monkeys and humans are susceptible and may become a source of the virus if they become infected. Tissues of infected primates can also serve as a source of infection to staff in laboratories or in import and quarantine facilities that handle primates.

Viral hemorrhagic fever begins with fever and muscle aches, and it can result in a relatively mild illness or lead to death. To date, there have been four known outbreaks of *Ebola* virus involving humans; two in Sudan (in 1976 and 1979) and two in Zaire (in 1976 and 1995). In most of the outbreaks of *Ebola* virus infection, the majority of cases occurred in hospital settings where inadequate medical supplies resulted in poor infection-control practices. There have been no confirmed human cases of *Ebola* virus hemorrhagic fever in the United States.

In Summary

- In crowds, basic sanitation practices, such as hand-washing and not touching your eyes, nose, and mouth, are essential.
- Always look into the immunization (vaccination) requirements of a country before any kind of travel. The site http://wonder.cdc.gov/wonder/prev-guid/m0025228/entire.htm details all of the different immunizations needed for travel both inside and outside the United States, as well as links to individual countries.
- Cruise ships must carry most of their own food and water, so there is a greater risk for contamination.

- In underdeveloped countries, either buy bottled water or boil any water you drink.
- Drinking untreated water, especially in the wild, leaves you open for infection.
- If you can't boil the water you get from a stream, then you can use water purification tablets that contain chlorine or iodine.
- *Ebola* illness, which is still quite rare, can be found in both humans and primates.

Chapter Seventeen

Bioterrorism—When Good Germs Go Bad

In the natural scheme of things, the number of helpful bacteria and fungi that can save human lives far outweighs the number that can take lives. In the unnatural scheme of things, however, we no longer can afford to ignore the possibility that germs can be used as weapons.

Biological material in the form of infectious agents or toxins has been developed, and, if used by terrorists, it is as effective as guns and bombs. On March 20, 1995, a radical Japanese group, Aum Shinrikyo (Supreme Truth), used a kind of nerve gas to attack unsuspecting people in Tokyo's subway system. After subsequent investigation into the attack, it was found that this same group had also experimented with and considered the use of botulism toxin and the organism that causes anthrax, *Bacillus anthracis,* as biological weapons.

The relative success of this attack and the continued acts of terrorist groups around the globe have caused many nations' leaders to become much more concerned about bioterrorism.

Is biological warfare something new?

The use of biological warfare is nearly as old as civilization itself. Here are just a few incidents involving biological weapons, according to the Center for Nonproliferation Studies (CNS):

1346–1347 A.D.:
> Mongols catapult corpses contaminated with the plague over the walls into Kaffa (Crimea), forcing besieged Genoans to flee.

1767:
> During the French and Indian Wars, the British give blankets that had been used to wrap British smallpox victims to hostile Indian tribes.

1916–1918:
> German agents use anthrax and the equine disease glander to infect livestock and feed for export to Allied troops.

1939: (Nomohan Incident)
> Japanese poison Soviet water supply with intestinal bacteria at Mongolian border.

1940:
> The Japanese drop rice and wheat mixed with plague-carrying fleas over China and Manchuria.

What is the strategy for using a biological agent for a terrorist attack?

Germs are a terrorist's biological weapons of choice for several different reasons: First, the amount of organic material required to cause significant harm is small and is therefore easy to carry and distribute, making it relatively simple to expose large numbers of people over a short span of time. Second, if an infectious agent is chosen for the attack, the harm could be spread among members of the population long after the initial attack occurred.

What biological agents are likely to be used?

Biological agents such as botulism toxin, the bacteria that cause anthrax and the plague, and the virus that causes smallpox are the ones experts on terrorism predict would most likely be used. The effect of each of these agents on humans varies from person to person, but all can result in serious and possibly long-lasting harm to an individual. We'll take a look at each of these agents in turn and discuss the damage each can inflict. By the time we're finished, you'll see exactly why these bugs could be so very dangerous in the wrong hands.

Botulism

Botulism toxin is a protein manufactured by certain members of *Clostridium botulinum* that have been infected with a bacterial virus. The toxin, usually released from the bacterium when the cell dies, is one of the most deadly nerve poisons known. One ounce (a little more than twenty-eight grams) of any one of them could kill the entire population of the United States. The toxin prohibits the electrical signals of nerves from traveling to the muscle tissue, thereby paralyzing the muscle.

Immediate treatment is necessary and consists of injection of botulism-specific anti-toxin (a mixture of antibodies known to block the effects of all known forms of botulism toxin) and breathing assistance. Without treatment, the ultimate outcome is respiratory arrest and probably death. Based upon the outcome of accidental cases of botulism poisoning (eating improperly canned food, for example), those affected who did not die required breathing assistance for as long as two months after exposure and treatment. Because botulism poisoning is relatively rare in the United States (at around 100 cases per year), the local supply of anti-toxin preparations is low and, if there were an outbreak, would be rapidly exhausted. Luckily, the effects of the toxin cannot be spread from person to person, as the toxin itself is not infectious.

Anthrax

Anthrax is a deadly disease that affects both humans and animals and is caused by *Bacillus anthracis,* a spore-forming bacterium found in soil. Because of its capacity to form spores under stress, the organism is particularly resilient. Naturally occurring anthrax can be a problem in certain parts of the world, including Asia, Africa, the Caribbean, Central and South America,

Eastern and southern Europe, and the Middle East. It is rare in the United States, with only 230 or so cases reported to the CDC over the last forty-plus years. None of the forms of anthrax disease are apparently transferred from person to person.

After infecting a person or animal, this bacterium produces deadly toxins. There can be at least three different results of this infection, depending upon where in the body the organism attaches and grows. The first and least deadly (with antibiotic treatment) is a skin infection known as cutaneous anthrax. This disease is most common among folks who work with animals or who handle animal hides, particularly hides from sheep and goats (the germ can be picked up in the animal's hair when an animal rolls in or stirs up dirt). Although this is the mildest illness caused by anthrax, without antibiotic treatment about 20 percent of those infected will die. The second most harmful form of the disease is intestinal anthrax, which is acquired from eating contaminated meat from animals that are infected with the bug or drinking water contaminated with the spores of the bug. Antibiotics also can help against this form of the disease, but even if they are used, intestinal anthrax is between 20 and 60 percent fatal.

The last and worst form of the disease is respiratory anthrax. Once the spores are inhaled, the disease kills approximately 90 percent of its victims. What makes this form of anthrax so deadly as a terrorist weapon is that it is easily dispersed into the air or water, since the spores are colorless, odorless, and tasteless. Respiratory anthrax is particularly dangerous because, at least initially, only flu-like symptoms appear. Within a few days, however, severe symptoms appear: Lungs fill with fluid and breathing becomes terribly difficult. But by this time, a person would likely have only one or two days to live, far too little time left for any known treatment to save him.

The vaccine that treats the cutaneous form of anthrax might be useful against the other forms. However, because of the inability to test the vaccine ethically against intestinal and respiratory anthrax, it is not known whether it can adequately protect individuals from these forms of the disease. Because of the rising significant risk to personnel that this organism represents, the U.S. military has, however, instituted an active immunization program.

Plague

Plague, known as the Black Death, is estimated to have killed 100 million people in the Middle East, Europe, and Asia during the sixth century. During the fourteenth century, it killed one-fourth to one-half the population of Europe. The plague, which is caused by the bacterium *Yersinia pestis,* is typically found within the fleas that feed upon various kinds of rodents. *Yersinia* is a bioterrorist's weapon of choice primarily because, similar to anthrax, it would be easy to disperse and has a high likelihood of killing about one-third of the victims in as little as three days. Additionally, the organism is highly infectious, particularly in what is known as the pneumonic form (where the lungs are affected), and a person with plague could easily infect others not originally exposed to the bug. Consequently, unlike anthrax, plague would spread from person to person among the population in a way similar to the naturally occurring plague outbreaks that happened centuries ago.

Smallpox

The virus *Variola* causes smallpox, a disease that can result in a 40 percent fatality rate. But even if one survives, *Variola* causes a long, debilitating illness, as well as possible disfigurement and/or blindness. The virus first multiplies in the mucosal tissue of the upper respiratory tract and can be spread by droplets of moisture from the infected person's mouth (before any skin lesions appear). As a consequence, this virus is highly contagious and can easily spread through a population even if only a few people are originally infected. One tiny drop of saliva from an infected person, generated simply by talking, is estimated to contain 1,000 more virus particles than are required to infect someone.

Evidence suggests that the disease has an ancient history; the mummy of Ramses V, a pharaoh who died about 1160 B.C. in Egypt, has smallpox scars. Historical accounts and more recent records indicate that smallpox has a terrible ability to kill and was responsible over the centuries for more deaths than bubonic plague, cholera, or yellow fever combined. More recently, it is estimated that between 1900 and 1979, over 500 million people in the world died from smallpox—an average of approximately 6 million people per year.

The virus infects only humans and therefore can be passed only from person to person. Therefore, it is not possible to remove the source of infection (the host), for example, eliminating rats that harbor the fleas that harbor plague organisms. Because of a massive vaccination effort by the WHO and other organizations, the entire planet was considered to be free of this virus in October of 1979. With the risk of harm from vaccination larger than the risk of encountering the virus, people are no longer being vaccinated, resulting in millions of people being vulnerable to smallpox.

Although the natural occurrence of the smallpox virus has disappeared, a few places keep the virus stored in case the need to fight smallpox arises in the future. Frozen laboratory stocks of live smallpox virus exist under *official* circumstances in two places: in maximum-containment laboratories at the CDC in Atlanta, Georgia, and at a facility in Moscow, Russia. An ongoing world-wide debate among scientists questions whether or not to destroy these remaining stocks of this virus. On one hand, some feel that these facilities would be easy targets for terrorists who could confiscate the virus and spread the disease to the general population. Others feel that stocks of this virus may secretly exist in other places within the former Soviet Union, Iraq, North Korea, and perhaps in other countries as well. Therefore, care must be taken not to eliminate the samples of smallpox held in the United States and Russia, just in case.

Don't Touch That Doorknob!

What can we do to protect ourselves?

There really is little an individual can do to avoid any terrorist attack, including a biological attack. Even if the disease could be rapidly diagnosed, it might not be possible to protect other individuals from the spread of infection. It would take an estimated two to three years to generate a viable smallpox vaccine (prepared from *Vaccinia* virus, a close relative to the smallpox virus), since the current supplies of this vaccine are low and it is not known precisely whether the ones that remain are still useful. There is also a possibility that any bacterial agents used in such an attack could be genetically altered to resist the effects of all known antibiotics. Evidence presented by Ken Alibek, an expert on biological weapons and former deputy chief of the Soviet Main Directorate Biopreparat, has proven that such agents do exist. As a consequence, health facilities would find antibiotic therapy of no use. Further, many medical personnel caring for patients would be at particular risk and would probably become infected themselves.

What is our government doing to prepare for a biological attack?

Our local, state, and national governments are maintaining an active vigil to identify terrorist groups and to assess their ability to stage an attack. Because this is a worldwide issue, an incredible and perhaps uncommon degree of cooperation among all governments is necessary to deal with the threat of biological attacks by terrorists.

252

In response to this threat, the U.S. government has established training procedures for all public-health personnel. In 1999, Congress assigned the CDC with the responsibility of overseeing the nation's preparedness against this particular terrorist threat. The CDC's mission is to coordinate the upgrade of all state and local public-health systems in regard to a response against a biological agent. The CDC has also been assigned the task of developing well-organized, interconnected communications systems at the federal level that could immediately respond should a biological attack occur. Over $120 million was allocated for these purposes.

The CDC has since established a laboratory system that can provide local agencies across the United States with the ability to identify suspected infectious agents rapidly. They have also created the Health Alert Network, a state-of-the-art telecommunications and computer network that links all local and state health departments throughout the United States. The many other precautions that should be taken include continued practice drills in local areas by medical and other personnel in handling such an emergency.

In Summary

- The potential for terrorists to use biological agents to cause harm is a reality.
- The biological agents most likely to be used by terrorists cause the diseases known as anthrax, botulism poisoning, plague, and smallpox.

- In a terrorist act, these biological agents would likely be distributed among a population via a municipal water supply or by aerosol in a confined area.
- Governments throughout the world are aware of the threat of bioterrorism.
- To stop terrorism, cooperative agreements among responsible nations of the world must be supported and encouraged.

Chapter Eighteen

Making Peace with the Germs Among Us

While microorganisms can be used to take lives, they are more commonly responsible for saving them. Entire industries are devoted to using germs to help us, from nutritional supplements to antibiotics to cleaning up oil spills. So why don't we detail some of the positive things these remarkable little critters can do?

No matter how helpful something is, in time somebody seems to find a way to use it to cause harm. Occasionally, the table turns and something bad is used to do good. Allow me again to introduce you to *Clostridium botulinum*, a bug previously described as producing a very dangerous toxin. Over the last several years, the botulism toxin's paralyzing effect has been used successfully to treat some people with debilitating medical disorders. After several years of study and clinical trials, in 1989 the Food and Drug Administration (FDA) approved the use of botulism toxin Type A (named Oculinum, also known as BoTox) for medical use to treat two conditions, blepharospasm and strabismus. Each of these maladies causes uncontrolled facial muscle contractions, resulting in continuous closure of the eyelid, or what may be more commonly known as "cross-eye" or "lazy eye," respectively. The toxin prevents these muscle contractions.

Because of its success in treating these diseases, the use of the botulism toxin to treat all kinds of neurological disorders, or dystonias, is under investigation. These conditions include neck and shoulder muscle contraction (spasmodic torticollis), clenching of the jaw muscles (oral mandibular dystonia), improper vocal cord contractions (spasmodic dysponia), as well as writers' and musicians' cramp. Applications of this toxin for treatment of facial tics, cerebral palsy spasms, and esophageal sphincter-muscle spasms are also under investigation. That's quite a lot of potential from a toxin so deadly.

Except for use against the eye disorders mentioned above, all other medicinal uses of the toxin are known as "off-label," which denotes clinical use by a licensed physician of a drug for a purpose not originally approved by the FDA, such as the use of aspirin to prevent heart attacks. The FDA approves drugs through a long-term clinical study to treat very specific ailments. When a drug licensed by the FDA for the treatment of "Y" is used by a licensed physician for the treatment of "X," this use is considered off-label. An additional off-label use of botulism toxin is involved in cosmetic surgery to eliminate facial wrinkles. This specific use is, however, not one the FDA particularly likes. In fact, in a November 18, 1994, Federal Register notice, the FDA denounced the promotion of the use of this still very dangerous toxin for cosmetic purposes.

Do many microorganisms help us?

Following is a list selected from information in *Foundations in Microbiology* and *Brock Biology of Microorganisms* of common items and their genesis in microorganisms.

Antibiotics (antibacterial substances)	Microbial Source
Amphotericin B	*Streptomyces* (bacterium)
Bacitracin	*Bacillus subtilis* (bacterium)
Cephalosporin	*Cephalosporium* (fungus)
Erythromycin	*Streptomyces* (bacterium)
Penicillins	*Penicillium chrysogenum* (fungus)
Tetracycline	*Streptomyces* (bacterium)

Vitamins (necessary for enzyme function)	Microbial Source
Riboflavin (dietary supplement)	*Ashbya gossypii* (fungus)
Vitamin B$_{12}$ (dietary supplement)	*Pseudomonas denitrificans* (bacterium)

Steroids (anti-inflammatory agents)	Microbial Source
Steroids (cortisone)	*Rhizopus* (fungus)

Food Additives and Amino Acids
(acidifiers, dietary supplements, flavor enhancers)

	Microbial Source
Acetic acid (many food and industrial uses)	*Acetobacter* (bacterium)
Citric acid (pharmaceuticals, foods)	*Aspergillus,* *Candida* (fungi)
Glutamic acid (flavor enhancer)	*Corynebacterium,* *Arthrobacter* (bacteria)
Lactic acid (acidifier)	*Lactobacillus* (bacterium)
Lysine (dietary supplement)	*Corynebacterium*
Xanthan (food stabilizer)	*Xanthomonas* (bacterium)

Various Chemicals
(solvents, blood expanders, absorbents)

	Microbial Source
Acetone (industrial solvent)	*Clostridium* (bacterium)
Butanol (industrial solvent)	*Clostridium* (bacterium)
Dextran (blood expander, absorbent)	*Klebsiella, Acetobacter* (bacteria)
Ethanol (industrial solvent)	*Saccharomyces* (fungus/yeast)
Glycerol (explosives)	Yeast

258

As you can see, microorganisms are used in a wide variety of ways. About 90 percent of the antibiotics used to treat bacterial infections are created from microorganisms, most of them bacteria. These bugs benefit us indirectly as well. Intense study of how these microorganisms function has led to the design of completely synthetic antibiotics in the laboratory, which may help combat microorganisms' increasing resistance to the effects of our present-day therapeutic drugs. Microorganisms are also used in food, such as yeast (a form of fungus) to make bread and to make beer in the brewing industry, and bacteria in milk that makes yogurt. The same goes for the production of cheese and buttermilk, and other nondairy products like sauerkraut, pickles, and a few kinds of sausage. All of these foods depend on microbes and their specific actions to make them what they are.

Not only do bacteria contribute to the creation of certain foods, they also produce supplements that are added to food. Aspartame, the artificial sweetener that is used in soft drinks and sugar-free food, is the combination of two amino acids, phenylalanine and glutamic acid, both of which are commercially produced by bacteria. Many foods do not have all of the different or the right amount of amino acids required for a healthy human. Again, good bacteria to the rescue: The amino acid lysine, necessary for our good health, is added as a food supplement, making these foods healthier.

Aren't all vitamins synthetically manufactured in laboratories?

Although we can make synthetically many of the substances that bacteria or fungi synthesize naturally, sometimes it is far too difficult and expensive to do so. In these cases, we recruit the germs themselves to make these chemically very complicated substances for us. A good example of this process is two highly chemically complex but critical vitamins required for our health: Vitamin B_{12} from *Pseudomonas denitrificans* (bacterium) and riboflavin from *Ashbya gossypii* (fungus). It is telling that an often bad germ like *Pseudomonas*—one that can cause eye infections from contaminated makeup or infect the exposed tissue of burn patients—may also be made useful.

Can any of these bugs be used for medical purposes other than production of antibiotics and supplements?

Streptoccocus, the genus of bacteria that causes strep throat and tissue destruction, also produces the enzyme streptokinase. This enzyme is used medically to dissolve blood clots and to thin blood. Additionally, this genus of bacteria has members that produce an enzyme that helps wounds to heal properly. But we aren't finished yet: There are a number of bacteria that produce an enzyme named hyaluronidase that is used to clean wounds—accidental or surgical—and to reduce or prevent adhesions, or heal tissue connections. And we still aren't finished: The fungus *Rhizopus nigricans* is used to convert bile chemicals to the very medically useful substance cortisone.

What about genetic engineering of these germs?

Laboratory strains of certain organisms are used to produce human substances, most commonly yeast and our old friend *E. coli.* So much has been discovered about how genes work that it is possible to have a human protein made inside a bacterium or yeast cell. Since we can grow billions of these cells at any one time, we can make as much of a particular protein as we need, a process that alone has saved many lives. For example, human insulin, a hormone found in extremely low concentrations in the blood, is essentially impossible to isolate. In the past (and currently, in some cases) people with insulin-dependent diabetes used insulin prepared from the blood of cows or horses (bovine or equine insulin), which is almost identical to human insulin in structure. But now, thanks to genetic engineering methods, human insulin made in yeast or *E. coli* is available to everyone.

This bacterium or yeast can also help produce erythropoietin, a protein necessary for the proper development of red blood cells that is present in minute amounts in blood. A person without kidneys is unable to produce this protein. Before the genetic manufacture of erythropoietin, such a person was required to receive timely doses of this protein that was isolated from other humans in order for red blood cells to mature and function properly. Because of genetic engineering, this protein is now made in cells in large quantity and is available to all who need it.

What is bioremediation?

Germs can be used to clean areas where toxic materials have been released. This process, known as bioremediation, is a rapidly growing industry. Examples include:

- Certain bacteria can degrade nitro-containing explosives and are used to clean up the gunpowder released from dismantled ammunition of all sorts.
- Scientists are examining how planting vegetation that attracts *Arthrobacter* bacteria can help clean oil spills on land.
- Almost all water-purification systems use germs to degrade solid waste and convert it to harmless substances.

Can the study of germs provide new explanations for old diseases?

Scientists are discovering that some infections may cause organic problems. Recent research data suggest the bacterium *Chlamydia pneumoniae* might be associated with heart disease in some individuals. The bacterium itself may not cause the damage, but rather the immune system's response to it in certain individuals may lead to tissue damage of the heart and associated blood vessels.

Reports in 1997 from British researchers revealed that men who suffered heart attacks were four times more likely to suffer an additional heart attack if their blood contained high levels of antibodies (the proteins produced by the immune system against infectious agents) against *Chlamydia*. If these men received an antibiotic, the risk was reduced to the same level as the men who had none of these antibodies present in their circulation. Following this study, investigators at the Ontario Cancer Institute and University of Toronto in Canada reported in 1999 that a similarity of certain *Chlamydia* proteins to human heart muscle might account for heart damage possibly caused by an immune response against the bug.

An analogous situation concerns that of rheumatic fever, a complication of *Streptococcus pyogenes* infection in some individuals. Heart damage can occur due to the type of immune response certain individuals generate against *S. pyogenes,* the bug that causes "strep" throat. Some people make very reactive antibodies against one of the bacterium's proteins, and these same antibodies can also react with human heart muscle. Since the immune system is designed to harm things that have antibodies attached to them, the heart muscle suffers the same fate.

On the basis of these and further studies, it might be possible one day to treat heart disease or other "naturally-occurring" diseases in certain people with antibiotics. Consequently, there is all the more reason to investigate all of these little critters and try to understand how they interact with us and we with them.

All in all, then, how do we find a way to live with microorganisms?

Most microorganisms are necessary in our lives, both directly and indirectly. So do not be overly concerned about the presence of these germs in your life. Use common sense and the simple but effective precautions outlined in this book to avoid the dangerous germs. Wash your hands often. Keep things around the house reasonably clean with soap and water. Pay attention to preparing food properly. Be reasonably prepared for any risky situation you may face, either through research or immunization. Try to keep in mind that our immune system exists to fight off many infections before we are in serious trouble. Good nutrition, exercise, and getting enough sleep will set the stage for combating any vicious bug that has the nerve to harm us. For those who may be more vulnerable to infections, take the reasonable precautions we've detailed and discuss any issue of concern with your physician.

For the majority of people, sterilizing your home or your body would not be healthy. Indiscriminate use of antibacterial substances has the potential to lead to the increase of some very strong and more harmful strains of germs. This overuse also kills the good germs, which we need to take up living space and compete for available nutrients and thereby reduce the chances of the bad guys getting the upper hand. That does not mean that you should not occasionally use such agents, such as diluted bleach, to help protect yourself from infectious germs or to kill the critters multiplying inside the garbage disposal. Just do not try continuously to eliminate every good and bad bug in your home.

Keep in mind that there is only so much a person can reasonably do to avoid an infectious illness. Stay up to date with recommended vaccinations. Pay attention to where you are and where you are going. What is your risk of contracting the *Ebola* virus in the United States? Essentially zero. But if you travel to Zaire and there happens to be an outbreak near you, the chances increase.

In the grand scheme of things, then, it doesn't matter how old you are, what you do for a living, where you live, where you travel, what you eat, what you drink, or to which race, creed, or gender you happen to belong. Germs are everywhere: overwhelmingly doing good things, and a few doing very bad things, but they are around us and within us, and are part of our daily lives. Do not be intimidated by them. Instead, find out more about them. You just might be glad you did.

Special Thanks

I wish to thank my editor, Dinah Dunn, for her unfailing interest, her hard work, her crisp and consistently accurate comments, her graceful ability to turn incomprehensible passages into clearly written statements, and for her remarkable skill in maintaining an appropriate focus throughout the text. Thank you also Byron Preiss and Jeanine Campbell at Byron Preiss Visual Publications, Inc. Additionally, I would like to thank all of the people at Warner Books who worked hard to bring this book to completion: My editor at Warner, Jackie Merri Meyer, Nina Poliseno, Diane Luger, Shasti O'Leary, Anna Maria Piluso, Harvey-Jane Kowal, Eric Wechter, Karen Thompson, Ann Schwartz, and Huy Duong.

I especially thank my wife, Mary Ellen, first for who she is, but also for her many important ideas, for her untiring willingness to discuss this work, and for her unwavering support and confidence in me. I would never have attempted to write the book had it not been for her.

I thank my children. First, Martha Elizabeth, for her consistent interest in my writing, for her not once complaining about relinquishing time on the computer in order that I could work longer, and for being who she is. And I thank Aaron and Rachel, now adults, for their interest and support, for being who they are, and for gently refusing to allow me to influence them to be who they are not.

I thank Martha Elizabeth's friends, Kondja, Kristen, and Lauren, for insisting that they be acknowledged because they so often had to listen to me talk about this book.

I thank Brigadier General H. W. Hise, USMC (Ret.) and his wife, Frances, for their help in collecting useful information and for asking pertinent text-related questions.

Last, I wish to thank my mother, Laura Belle Roberts Brown, for sharing with me her insatiable curiosity about life, and for having taught me that to learn something new is always worthwhile.

Glossary

Acidic Any substance that releases a positive electrically charged hydrogen ion in solution is acidic (the substance on release of the hydrogen ion subsequently acquires a negative electrical charge). Acid solutions have a sour taste (like lemon juice). When an acid, such as hydrochloric acid (HCl), mixes with a base such as sodium hydroxide (NaOH), a salt will form (as in the formation of table salt, sodium chloride—NaCl).

Adenoids The adenoids are lymphoid tissue regions of the upper respiratory tract within the nasal cavity at the back of the throat that are involved in immune responses. During childhood, the adenoids may become swollen and can obstruct breathing.

Adrenal glands The adrenal glands, of which there are two in humans, lie atop each kidney. There are two regions within each adrenal gland, the medulla and the cortex. The medulla produces the hormone adrenaline (epinephrine), which is important during the "fight or flight" response in an emergency because it stimulates the breakdown of stored carbohydrate that results in the release of a burst of energy. The cortical region is responsible for producing approximately thirty different kinds of steroids necessary for regulation of many different cellular functions. One of these compounds, cortisol, regulates the metabolism of carbohydrate, fats, and proteins in the body.

Aerosol Microscopic solid or liquid particles that are tiny enough to be suspended as a gaseous medium. Fog and smoke are naturally occurring aerosols; when we sneeze, we produce an aerosol. Aerosols containing infectious agents generated by an infected individual can lead to transmission of diseases from one person to another.

Aflatoxin Complex chemical compounds released by the fungal organisms *Aspergillus flavus* and *Aspergillus parasiticus* that are highly toxic and carcinogenic (cancer-causing) in animals. These fungi usually grow most commonly on moist nuts and grains, but the toxins produced by them can be found in milk products as well. The Environmental Protection Agency of the United States (EPA) has established allowable action levels of aflatoxins in foodstuffs, limited to 20 parts per billion in feed and nut products and 0.5 parts per billion in milk.

Algae Algae are eukaryotic microorganisms that with some exceptions are capable of photosynthesis. Normally single celled, some algae can become large, many-celled plant-like structures (kelp and seaweed). These organisms live primarily in freshwater and oceans and together with photosynthetic bacteria produce most of the earth's atmospheric oxygen.

Glossary

Alkaline Any substance that scavenges hydrogen ions from solution or neutralizes hydrogen ions through a reaction to form water is alkaline (base, or basic) or has a negative electrical charge. For example, ammonia (NH_3) is a weak base because it scavenges hydrogen ions from solution and forms ammonium (NH^{4+}) ions. Like strong acids, strong bases can cause severe burns of the skin.

Allergies Allergies are caused by a bad immune reaction to any substance that may be inhaled, touched, or ingested that the body recognizes as potentially harmful. Symptoms of an allergic reaction may include one or more of the following: redness and warmth at the surface of the skin, increased mucus flow, itching, a rash, raised bumps (hives), tissue swelling, breathing difficulties, coughing, sneezing or a "runny" nose. Mild and relatively harmless allergies lead to sneezing, runny noses, and perhaps itching, while severe allergies, such as asthma, can lead to lung damage. A severe allergic reaction against bee venom can lead to a condition known as anaphylactic shock (rapid loss of blood pressure and organ failure) and can be fatal if not treated.

Amino acids Organic compounds that are composed of a carboxyl group (COOH) and an amino group (NH_2) and sometimes additionally contain sulfur (S). Amino acids are the building blocks used by a cell to make proteins. There are twenty amino acids required for all living cells on earth to survive; human adults require eight of the amino acids, and growing children require nine amino acids (together known as the essential amino acids) to be provided in the diet. Human cells can synthesize the remainder.

Antibiotic Any substance produced by one microorganism that kills or inhibits the growth of a different microorganism. Examples of antibiotics are penicillin, erythromycin, and streptomycin. An example of a synthetic antibiotic is ciprofloxacin.

Antibiotic resistance The ability of bacteria to combat the effects of an antibiotic. This resistance is due to the presence of an enzyme that destroys the drug, to the ability to pump the drug out of the cell, to the lack of a transport mechanism to bring the drug into the cell, or to the presence of a protein that binds to and inactivates the drug. In most cases resistance occurs through the acquisition of new genetic information in the form of a plasmid, which is a source of genetic information (genes) completely independent of the chromosome that is composed of double-stranded, closed-circular DNA. Plasmids can be acquired by a bacterial cell from the environment or by transfer among similar bacterial cells.

Antibodies Antibodies are proteins of different sizes (depending on the particular kind of antibody, such as IgM or IgG, for example) produced by B-lymphocytes during an immune response against foreign substances or microorganisms that invade the body. Antibodies are special proteins that can bind specifically to a particular shape that is present on other molecules. Antibodies circulate within the bloodstream and lymph system and can enter the tissues, and, once within the blood or tissues, antibodies can specifically interact with proteins or sugars or whole organisms such as bacteria and viruses that may be present. This reaction can lead to the inactivation and/or removal of toxins and microorganisms from the body. We depend upon antibodies to protect us from infectious diseases.

Antifungal agents Chemical compounds used for therapeutic purposes that either retard the growth of or kill a fungus that causes disease. Examples of antifungal agents include Tinactin (used for treatment of athlete's foot), miconazole, and nystatin. Because fungal cells are so similar in function to human cells, antifungal agents can be toxic to humans and other animals.

Antigen Any substance that can bind specifically to (react with) an antibody molecule (meaning that the binding site of the antibody specifically associates with a shape present on the antigen). Antigens include proteins, sugar polymers, bacterial cells, and viruses. Very small chemical structures (aspenicillin, for example) are not considered to be antigens. The name is derived from the term *antibody generating*. Although they are able to interact with an antibody, some antigens cannot generate an immune response. Antigens that generate immune responses (through antibody production or cell killing) are termed *immunogens*. Thus, all immunogens are antigens, but only some antigens are immunogens.

Anti-inflammatory Any agent that either blocks the action of or inhibits the production of substances that cause inflammatory response symptoms, such as dilation of the capillary beds, increased mucus secretion and fluid (lymph) accumulation in tissues, or constriction of smooth muscle. Histamine is an inflammatory substance that is produced in some allergic reactions. Anti-histamine is an example of an anti-inflammatory substance that serves to control the effects of this substance.

Antimicrobial agents Any substances that kill or weaken microorganisms. Although antifungal agents are also antimicrobials, the microorganisms usually associated with the term *antimicrobial* most often involve bacteria and viruses. Bleach is an antimicrobial agent, as are certain formulations of iodine and other chemical compounds (such as common soap).

Antiviral Any substance that is used therapeutically to lower the activity of a virus substantially. All current antiviral agents do not completely eliminate the virus, but do significantly interfere with replication of the virus, thus lowering the number of virus particles available for further infection of cells. Examples of antiviral agents used for therapy include aclyovir (for the herpes virus infection) and amantadine (for influenza virus infections).

Asexual reproduction The generation of cellular offspring in the absence of a fusion of nuclei. Simple division of these cells produces new individuals (cells). Asexual reproduction takes place by cellular budding from a parent system, by spore formation (as with fungi), or by binary fission. The resulting cell develops as a new individual.

Binary fission The process that all bacteria, as well as some eukaryotic cells such as fungi, undergo when reproducing. The process is an asexual form of reproduction, since two new cells are produced in the absence of any "joining" of genetic material from two different sources. A bacterium, after almost doubling in size, replicates (makes an exact duplicate of itself) the chromosome, and synthesis of a new cell wall occurs. The cytoplasmic contents of the cell are equally divided as this cell splits to become two identical, independent cells.

Carcinogenic Anything that is capable of causing cancer, the condition of non-regulated cell division.

Carrier The term, in the sense of pathogenic microbiology, refers to an animal that does not exhibit specific disease symptoms yet harbors and is capable of transferring an infectious agent to a different animal.

Cell division The process that occurs when a single cell enlarges, doubles the amount of genetic material by replication of the cell's DNA, and then divides in half to produce two new (daughter) cells. Each daughter cell contains the identical amount and kind of DNA and cytoplasmic components.

Cell walls In bacteria, the cell wall is the general non-chemical term used to describe the rigid, cross-linked structure made of sugars and amino acids that surrounds almost all species of bacterial cells. The cell wall provides protection from rupture of the delicate membrane (plasma membrane) that encloses the cell's contents (cytoplasm). If not for the presence of the cell wall in bacteria, the plasma membrane could easily rupture due to the cell's internal water pressure.

Cellular lysis The process of plasma membrane rupture that results in release of all materials from the cytoplasm of a cell, and thus results in the death of the cell.

Cephalosporin antibiotics Complex antibacterial chemical compounds produced by the mold *Cephalosporium*.

Chromosome The complex chemical component composed of two individual strands of deoxyribonucleic acid (DNA) inside a cell that contains the cell's fundamental genetic information (genes). Each strand is wound around the other in a special helix, known as a DNA helix, that resembles a spiral. Bacteria have only one chromosome, which is arranged as a closed circle that contains the entire genetic information (genome) for the bacterium. All other living cells on earth have their genome represented by more than one chromosome (humans, for example, have forty-six). Viruses also have genetic material in the form of either DNA or RNA, but this material is not referred to as a chromosome but instead as the genome of the virus.

Chronic disease A disease that is continuously present. An *acute disease* occurs but then disappears after a period of time. High blood pressure (hypertension) is a chronic disease, whereas the common cold is an acute disease.

276

Cilia Hair-like external structures composed of tubulin that extend from the surface of protozoa and some eukaryotic cells. Certain cells (like those in airways) of higher forms of life (like humans) may also have cilia. Ciliated cells of the trachea, for example, sweep mucus up from the lungs. In protozoa, cilia are used to propel the microorganism.

Colony A bacterial colony is a group of identical cells that arise through cell division from a single parent cell.

Contagious A disease is contagious if it can be transmitted from one individual to another (one host to another) by direct or indirect contact with the person who is infected with the organism that causes the disease. Such a disease may also be called a communicable infectious disease. The common cold is a contagious disease and can be acquired from another person who has a cold—by inhalation of virus after the infected person sneezes, for example.

Contamination/contaminate This term refers to the process whereby microbial organisms or other impurities are present within food or water or upon surfaces. Food and water exposed to animal waste can become contaminated with harmful microorganisms.

Cross-contamination The series of events that can occur when an infectious agent on an object is transferred from the object to a clean surface by physical interaction. Placing pathogen-contaminated meat on a cutting board and then chopping vegetables on this board before washing the board can lead to cross-contamination of the vegetables.

Cultured Cultured cells are cells that are allowed to live and divide within containers of some type (tubes, bottles, or dishes) under defined conditions in the laboratory. Culture material may be liquid or semi-solid and will usually contain all of the nutrients necessary for the cells to live and to divide.

Cutaneous/subcutaneous vascular lesions Broken or disrupted blood vessels that occur within (cutaneous) or beneath (subcutaneous) the layers of skin tissue. If one grasps a patch of skin on the arm with the thumb and forefinger and pulls straight upward, the space underneath the fold, near the muscle tissue, is subcutaneous. This region lies above the muscle tissue and beneath the skin layers.

Cyst Any type of fluid-filled or fatty structure underneath the skin that is surrounded by tissue. This term (sometimes the term *spore* is referred to as a form of protozoa) is also used to describe a dormant but viable and environmentally resistant stage of a protozoan's life cycle (as found in the life cycles of *Giardia* and *Cryptosporidium*).

Dander The bits of hair, fluff, and particles that are shed from living creatures.

Dermis The deep layer beneath the epidermis that is composed of dense connective tissue. The dermis separates the skin from the muscle tissue underneath.

Extensive tearing of the dermis can occur when the skin is stretched too far such as in pregnancy, when the abdomen may acquire stretch marks. Separation of the epidermis from the dermis due to abrasion can cause a blister.

Detergent Most commonly synthesized from hydrocarbons (oily, non-polar compounds) isolated from crude oil, a detergent also contains either an acidic or basic polar (electrically charged) group that easily ionizes and thereby attracts water molecules. Detergents with negative charges on one end are known as anionic detergents. Those with positive ends are known as cationic detergents. The presence of both polar and non-polar regions allows detergents to enhance the cleaning power of solvents.

Disease outbreak A disease that first occurs as a focus among a few individuals and then spreads rapidly to infect a larger segment of the population. An outbreak of shigellosis or *E. coli* O157:H7 infection may occur within a local population were there to be bacterially contaminated drinking water at a day-care center, for example. A widespread outbreak that involves many, many people would be termed an epidemic. A worldwide outbreak would be termed a pandemic (such as the flu pandemic that occurred during World War I).

DNA The name of the chemical and the molecule made of connections (covalent bonds) between individual DNA compounds known as *deoxyribonucleotides* from which genes are made.

Dust mites The house dust mite (*Dermatophagoides pteronyssinus*) is an eight-legged microscopic insect that is distantly related to spiders. This tiny insect feeds on dead skin cells and most commonly lives in bedding and carpet. Material deposited by the house dust mite is considered responsible for the majority of allergic reactions in the world.

Emerging disease One that is only presently increasing in incidence within a given region of the world. Although the disease may have been identified in the past, the rise in status to an emerging disease results from the increase in incidence of that disease in a given region. For example, encephalitis caused by West Nile virus is an emerging disease within the temperate regions of Europe and North America (emerging in 1999 in the northeastern United States). *Ebola* virus emerged in recent years to cause disease in Africa.

Encephalitis Any inflammation of brain tissue usually caused by an infection of the tissue differing from the condition meningitis (which is an inflammation of the membranes that surround the brain and spinal cord) in that it specifically affects this area of the nervous system. Typically caused by a virus transmitted by the bite of a mosquito that previously bit an infected individual, bacteria and poisons encountered in the environment can also cause this condition. Examples of viruses that can cause this condition are the West Nile and St. Louis encephalitis virus (which can include several different kinds of viruses as an encephalitis-causing virus group).

Endemic The regularly found presence of an organism, disease, behavior, or situation within a given location. Something is said to be endemic when it is very common to a particular area and part of the general conditions. Fast-food restaurants are endemic to the United States; *E. coli* bacteria are endemic to the human intestinal tract.

Enzyme An organic catalyst made of protein that causes chemical reactions to occur within a cell. Just as any chemical catalyst functions, an enzyme lowers the energy of activation required for a chemical reaction to occur.

Epidermis The outermost layer of the skin of an animal and the first protective obstacle foreign organisms or substances must breach in order to invade the body. In humans, the epidermis consists mainly of cells named keratinocytes (they are filled with the protein keratin). These cells migrate to the surface from the mid-epidermal region. By the time the cells reach the surface they are dead and are sloughed off over time (called desquamation).

Eukaryote Cells that are unicellular or multicellular organisms with the DNA inside each cell completely surrounded by a special membrane. This intracellular membrane-bound structure with DNA inside is known as a nucleus. An example of an eukaryotic cell within a many-celled organism would be all of the cells within a human. A similar example for a single-celled organism would be the protozoan *Plasmodium,* the organism that causes malaria.

Fetus The stage of the developing human or animal in utero before birth when all major organs have formed. In the human, this stage extends from the ninth week of pregnancy until birth. A human embryo is the developmental stage that extends from two weeks after fertilization until the end of the eighth week of pregnancy.

Food-borne Associated with food as the source. A food-borne illness is one that is contracted from food of some sort.

Fungi Many-celled or single-celled eukaryotic microorganisms that belong to the *Eumycota* (true fungi), a classification group that includes all mildews, molds, mushrooms, and yeasts. They can reproduce either sexually or asexually, and although they resemble plants, they do not produce food by photosynthesis. Most fungi obtain nutrients by decomposition of dead organic matter. The single-celled fungi are known as yeasts, the filamentous fungi are known as molds, and those fungi that join together to form visible fleshy fruiting structures are known as mushrooms or puffballs. All fungi except for yeasts grow as tube-like branched filaments. A mycosis is a disease caused by a fungus.

Fungicide Any substance that when applied results in the death of a fungus.

Gastrointestinal The various regions of the digestive tract, which consist of the esophagus, stomach, small intestine (divided into the duodenum, jejunum, and ileum), and the colon (large intestine).

Glossary

Genome All of the genetic information available to an organism. A virus genome may be a short piece of single-stranded RNA. The *E. coli* genome is a single chromosome of double-stranded DNA that contains approximately 9.3 million deoxyribonucleotides. A human's genome (present in each egg and sperm cell) consists of twenty-three individual chromosomes of double-stranded DNA that determine everything physiologically about a person.

Germicide Any chemical that can kill bacteria and viruses.

Gram stain procedure Developed by Christian Gram in 1884, this process involves the use of colored dyes, crystal violet and safranin or fuschin, in addition to ethanol and iodine added in different stages to stain bacterial cells differentially. The individual staining properties of bacterial cells determine whether they are gram-positive or gram-negative bacteria. Gram-positive bacteria stain purple, while gram-negative bacteria stain red to pink.

HEPA filter High-efficiency particle-arresting filter. These filters, used in home-filtering units, are often used to prevent exposure to microscopic organisms, pollen, and mold spores.

Immune system A complex organization of circulating and organ-associated cells and products secreted by these cells that can eliminate microorganisms or foreign molecules (such as a protein toxin) from the body. It is this system that is activated whenever we have an infection, are vaccinated, or have an allergic reaction. The bone marrow, spleen, lymph nodes, thymus, lymphocytes, antibody molecules, and other cellular products are all part of this specific defense system. All vertebrates (animals with a backbone) possess an immune system, including the ancient animal the shark.

Immunization Immunization, or vaccination, refers to the process of introducing non-harmful forms of disease-causing foreign material into an animal in order to induce a specific, long-lived, and protective immune response against the disease caused by an infectious microorganism. With an immunization, the individual animal is normally protected from future potentially harmful effects due to exposure to the particular disease-causing agent or organisms that may be later encountered in the life of the animal.

Intubation The process of inserting a tube into a canal or hollow organ, such as when an endotracheal tube is inserted into the trachea to allow unimpeded passage of air into the lungs during anesthesia.

Keratin A highly water-insoluble protein produced by certain skin (epidermis) epithelial cells known as keratinocytes. The majority of the cells of the epidermis are keratinocytes. This protein, also present in the tissue of nails, feathers, hair, and hooves, provides a waterproof layer that helps to prevent entrance of foreign material into the body.

Latent condition A dormant state that certain viruses, commonly of the herpes virus family (varicella-zoster and herpes simplex virus Type I, for example) can assume inside a cell. The condition can reverse and the virus can become active again. An example of these conditions is the dormant virus condition that occurs after varicella-zoster (chickenpox) infection, that can revert to an active infection after many years of inactivity and lead to the skin disease known as shingles.

Lymph node Small, usually oval-shaped structures located along lymphatic vessels and connected to both lymphatic and blood vessels that contain mature lymphocytes. Immune responses against bacteria, viruses, and foreign particles occur within lymph nodes and provide activated lymphocytes to the bloodstream, resulting in removal of bacteria and foreign particles from the body.

Meningitis An inflammation of one or more of the three membranes (the tissues) that surround the brain. Many different viruses or bacteria may cause this inflammation, one or more familiar causes being the bug *Neisseria meninigiditis.*

Microflora Either plants or microorganisms that live in a given area that are invisible to the naked eye. The general reference for all plants, flora, may also refer to bacteria. Bacterial flora or microbial flora are terms most often used to describe bacteria that are normally found living within the intestines of animals (gut flora).

285

Micron A mathematical term that represents one-millionth of the length of one meter. Also called *Micrometer.*

Mildew Any area of fungal growth (usually light green or black) that can appear (most commonly under damp conditions) on books, clothing, leather, and other surfaces. Although this term is used most frequently in reference to fungi, in actuality mildews are specific plant diseases.

Mold Fungi that do not look like mushrooms. *Mildew* is a similar term used to describe certain fungi (on books, clothing, and old leather, for example), but mildews are actually plant diseases.

Mucosal tissues All openings from the human body to the external environment are lined with specialized cells that form mucosal tissue. There are different kinds and slightly different functions of mucosal tissue that are associated with specific locations. These tissues are the oral, gastrointestinal, urogenital, and respiratory mucosa. Mucosal cells, regardless of location, produce the relatively sticky substance, mucus, that constantly bathes the inner surfaces of these openings and functions to trap microorganisms and helps to prevent attachment, growth, and entrance of these microorganisms into the body.

Mucus The slightly viscous, relatively sticky fluid substance secreted by mucosal tissue that constantly bathes the surface of all mucosal tissue that faces the openings to the environment. The specific contents of mucus differ for the different mucosal tissue involved, but there will always be present a collection of various ions and proteins that protect the tissue surface. The flow of mucus often traps and removes microorganisms that may have entered the exposed area.

Mutation In general terms, a mutation is any change or alteration of any system or process. In the context of this book, a mutation is any change or alteration of genetic information within a living organism. If the change of genetic information alters how the organism looks, behaves, or survives, the mutation may be readily apparent in offspring from that organism.

Mutualism Any mutually beneficial relationship between two species. For example, intestinal bacteria, such as *E. coli,* that live within the human colon derive nutrition from the association and, in turn, provide vitamin K and B-complex vitamins to the human.

Nasopharyngeal The area in the upper area of the pharynx (throat) most closely associated with the back of the nose.

Nosocomial infection Any infection that is acquired by a person after the person was admitted to a health-care facility. Although the term usually refers to an infection acquired by a patient, it is also used to describe an infection acquired by health-care personnel within the facility.

Nucleus A membrane-bound, internal structure within all eukaryotic cells. All of the chromosomes (made of DNA) within the cell are contained and separated from the other parts of the cell by a special membrane known as the nuclear membrane that completely envelops the area surrounding the chromosome. The presence of this membrane provides a barrier that separates all other cellular contents from the DNA and controls movement of selected molecules back and forth across the membrane.

Oropharyngeal The area of the pharynx most closely associated with the back of the mouth.

Parasite Any organism that lives at the expense of a different organism, does not provide the host any benefit, and may cause harm to the host.

Pathogen/pathogenic Any microorganism that can cause a disease in a different organism. For example, *Staphylococcus* is a human pathogen because this bacterium can cause disease in humans. Thus, *S. aureus* is a pathogenic bacterium.

Petri plate A flat-bottomed, circular, walled, shallow dish with a larger, shallower dish that serves as a lid. The Petri plate is used for semi-solid nutrient medium (agar) culture of bacteria and for liquid tissue cultures.

Pharynx The part of the throat that directs air into the trachea (the tube connected to the bronchial tubes, which lead to the lungs) or food and liquid into the esophagus (the tube that leads to the stomach).

Photosynthesis The process that most plants and some algae use to derive energy from sunlight. Light energy from the sun in the form of small packets known as photons is used to split water into its component parts, hydrogen and oxygen. The breakdown of water results in a release of chemical energy that is used to convert carbon dioxide into sugar, which the organism uses as food.

Plasma membrane This membrane consists of two closely associated layers, each of which is composed of fat and protein molecules that completely surround the internal contents of all cells, and separate the cytoplasm (all of the cellular contents enclosed by this membrane) from the outside environment.

Pneumonia A chronic or acute disease of the lungs due to inflammation that results from a bacterial or viral infection or chemical irritants. As a result, the ability to breathe properly and to obtain oxygen into the blood can be severely impaired.

Pollen The material produced by the male part of a flower that fertilizes the female part of other flowers of the same kind and results in seed production by the plant. Pollen is released by flowering plants.

Pore size Refers to the actual dimensions of the pore. If the pore is round, this dimension will be the diameter; if the pore is irregular or rectangular, the pore size will be the longest dimension. In practical use, the pore size reflects the lower limit in size an object can be in order to pass through the pore.

Prokaryote Microorganisms that do not contain an intracellular structure known as a nucleus. The DNA of a prokaryote is not surrounded by a selective membrane and is therefore exposed to the cytoplasm of the cell.

Prophylaxis Prophylaxis ("to guard against," "to protect") is the process used to prevent occurrence of disease. For example, a recommended prophylactic measure during "flu season" includes frequent hand-washing.

Protozoa Very small, unicellular eukaryotic, animal-like microorganisms of great diversity in size, shape, and function. The internal structures of these tiny microorganisms exhibit many of the functions that organs and tissue cells perform in higher, more complicated forms of life.

Quaternary ammonium compounds These compounds have a nitrogen atom with four chemical groups attached to it. This chemical arrangement causes the nitrogen atom to assume a permanent positive electrical charge with the chemical name of ammonium.

Rabies virus Cause of the disease known as rabies, this virus is a member of the rhabdovirus family and uses RNA as its fundamental genetic material (genome). Highly infectious and extremely dangerous, this virus can be easily transmitted through a bite or an already existing wound via the saliva of an infected warm-blooded animal (bats, raccoons, cats, and dogs, for example). Without proper treatment (injection of anti–rabies virus antibody and subsequent vaccination with rabies-virus proteins) the infection can cause severe and fatal neurological damage in humans as well as animals.

Replication The process by which genetic material, an organism, or a cell reproduces or makes an exact copy of itself.

RNA Ribonucleic acid, or RNA, is a large molecule made of connections (covalent bonds) between individual components known as ribonucleotides. Three different kinds of RNA inside a living cell are required for protein synthesis. Ribosomal RNA is a structural part of the cellular machinery (ribosome) used for making cell proteins. Messenger RNA contains information that chemically instructs the ribosome to place the building blocks (amino acids) in the correct order to make a particular protein. Transfer RNA carries the amino acids necessary for protein synthesis to the ribosome.

Sebum The substance produced by special glands in the skin known as sebaceous glands that is a mixture of different oils. Along with perspiration, these oils moisten and protect the skin.

Sepsis A systemic illness (poisoning) caused by an infection, toxic product of the infectious agent, or the body's response to the infection.

Spore form Bacteria in the two genera *Bacillus* and *Clostridium* can form an endospore (a spore form). The endospore is a dormant, thick-walled body that forms within the bacterial cell under extreme environmental stress (lack of nutrients or water). Some bacterial endospores can exist for thousands of years, only to become active again when environmental conditions improve.

Sterile/sterilization The process used to cause something to become devoid of all microorganisms. One common method of sterilization is to expose an object to a temperature of 121 degrees Celsius for fifteen minutes. If the object melts at that temperature, as an alternative procedure, high-energy radiation (gamma rays) may be used instead. For the purpose of this book, "sterile" does not refer to the inability to bear offspring.

Strain A group of organisms of the same species with unique, inheritable genetic traits that distinguish the group from other groups within the same species. Members of the *E. coli* O157:H7 strain of bacteria are unique members of the *coli* species of the genera *Escherichia* because of unique genetic material that enables this particular organism to produce harmful toxins.

Sulpha (sulfa) drugs Chemical compounds known collectively as sulfonamides that are used to treat bacterial infections.

Systemic Used to describe a process or the distribution of something throughout a system rather than within a localized area of the body. If an infection is systemic, the infection is present throughout the body of an organism. If a drug is systemic, the drug is distributed throughout the organism.

Tick A kind of insect, known as an arthropod, that has a segmented body, jointed legs, and, usually, a body shell. Ticks are parasites that live off the blood of their host. As a result, ticks can transmit various harmful bacterial, viral, and protozoan diseases (including Rocky Mountain spotted fever and Lyme disease) to animals, including humans.

Trivalent vaccine A vaccine that contains at least three different substances that are used for immunization (vaccination). The substances may be different proteins from the same organism, individual proteins from three different organisms, or three different organisms (active but attenuated, or non-active).

Unpasteurized Any food item (milk, in particular) that has not been subjected to a specific temperature for a specific length of time required for pasteurization. These temperatures and times are 71.6 degrees Celsius for at least 15 seconds (flash pasteurization), 62.9 degrees Celsius for at least 30 minutes (low-temperature, long-time pasteurization), or 87.8 degrees Celsius for 3 seconds (ultra-high-temperature treatment). Although pasteurized products are not sterile, pasteurization kills pathogens commonly found in milk (such as *Mycobacterium bovis,* one of the causes of human tuberculosis) and greatly lowers the number of organisms that spoil, or sour, milk.

Urethra The tube through which urine travels from the urinary bladder to the outside of the body, where it is emptied.

Vaccine/vaccination Any preparation that contains a harmless part of or form of bacterium, virus, or protozoan that is given to a person to stimulate the immune system to produce a response and protect the person from the disease caused by the bacterium, virus, or protozoan.

Vegetative cell A cell that divides into two cells by replicating the genetic material and splitting the cytoplasm between the two cells that appear. Also used to describe a conversion from a dormant form of a cell or organism (an endospore in bacteria or an oocyst in protozoa) into a fully functional, active cell or microorganism.

Virus A non-living but infectious biological entity that consists of genetic material in the form of either DNA or RNA. Visible only under an electron microscope, a virus infects an individual cell and can reproduce only inside the living host cell. Examples include influenza Type A, the virus that causes the flu; varicella-zoster, the virus that causes chicken pox; and *Bacteriophage lambda,* a virus that infects *E. coli*.

Vitamins Organic chemical compounds (other than amino acids) that are necessary for the proper action of various enzymes and bodily processes. Vitamin K, for example, is required in order for blood to clot effectively.

Certain B-complex vitamins are required for the exchange of amino groups among various amino acids and to prevent the disease pernicious anemia (lack of vitamin B_{12}).

Zoonosis Any infectious disease that can be transmitted from an animal to a human.

Resources

Books

Alberts, B.; D. Bray; J. Lewis; M. Raf; K. Roberts; and J. D. Watson, 1994, *Molecular Biology of the Cell,* third edition, Garland Publishing, Inc.

Atlas, R. M., 1995, *Principles of Microbiology,* first edition, Mosby-Year Book, Inc.

Atlas, R. M., 1995, *Microorganisms in Our World,* first edition, Mosby-Year Book, Inc.

Black, J. G., *Microbiology: Principles and Explorations,* 1999, fourth edition, Prentice Hall.

Goldsby, R. A.; T. J. Kindt; and B. A. Osborne, 2000, *Kuby Immunology,* fourth edition, W. H. Freeman and Co.

Ingraham, J. L., and C. A. Ingraham, 2000, *Introduction to Microbiology,* second edition, Brooks/Cole.

Janeway, C. A.; P. Travers; M. Walport; and J. D. Capra, 1999, *Immunobiology: The Immune System in Health and Disease,* fourth edition, Elsevier Science, Ltd./Garland Publishing.

Jensen, M. M.; D. N. Wright; and R. A. Robison, 1997, *Microbiology for the Health Sciences,* fourth edition, Prentice Hall.

Madigan, M. T.; J. M. Martinko; and J. Parker, 2000, *Brock Biology of Microorganisms,* ninth edition, Prentice Hall.

Nester, E. W.; C. E. Roberts; N. N. Pearsall; D. G. Anderson; and M. T. Nester, 1998, *Microbiology: A Human Perspective,* second edition, Wm. C. Brown, McGraw-Hill.

Prescott, L. M.; J. P. Harley; and D. A. Klein, 1999, *Microbiology,* fourth edition, Wm. C. Brown, McGraw-Hill.

Snyder, L., and W. Champness, 1997, *Molecular Genetics of Bacteria,* first edition, American Society for Microbiology.

Starr, C., and R. Taggart, 1992, *Biology: The Unity and Diversity of Life,* sixth edition, Wadsworth Publishing Co.

Talaro, K. P., and A. Talaro, 1999, *Foundations in Microbiology,* third edition, The McGraw-Hill Companies.

Tortora, G. J.; B. R. Funke; and C. L. Case, 1998, *Microbiology: An Introduction,* sixth edition, Benjamin/Cummings Publishing Co.

Volk, W. A., and J. C. Brown, 1997, *Basic Microbiology,* eighth edition, Addison-Wesley Educational Publishers, Inc.

World Wide Web Sites

Allergy and Immunology Sites on WebCrawler.com at http://www.webcrawler.com/health/diseases_and_conditions/allergies_and_immunology/?search=dust+mites32.

American Association of Immunologists: www.aai.org

American Society of Microbiology (ASM): www.asm.org

American Academy of Allergy and Immunology: www.aaaai.org

American Society for Microbiology—Microbes: www.microbe.org

Center for Food Safety and Applied Nutrition (CFSAN): www.cfsan.fda.gov

Centers for Disease Control and Prevention (CDC): www.cdc.gov

Centers for Disease Control and Prevention, The ABC's of Safe and Healthy Child Care: www.cdc.gov/ncidod/hip/abc/contents.htm

Centers for Disease Control and Prevention, Recommendations for Travelers' Vaccinations: www.cdc.gov/travel/vaccinat.htm

Centers for Disease Control and Prevention, Travel: www.cdc.gov/travel

Centers for Disease Control and Prevention, Food-borne Infections: www.cdc.gov/ncidod/dbmd/diseaseinfo/foodborne infections_g.htm

Child Care: National Child Care Information Center (NCCIC): www.nccic.org

Child-Care Licensure, State by State: National Resource Center for Health and Safety in Child Care at http://nrc.uchsc.edu/states.html

Choosing Child Care: National Child Care Information Center at nccic.org/cctopics/choosecc.html

Common Cold Fact Sheet: National Institutes of Health, National Institute of Allergy and Infectious diseases (NIAID) at www.niaid.nih.gov/factsheets/cold.htm

Consumer Advice: Food and Food Safety, Food and Drug Administration/Center for Food Safety and Applied Nutrition at vm.cfsan.fda.gov/~lrd/advice.html

Department of Health and Human Services: www.os.dhhs.gov

Disaster Preparedness: Federal Emergency Management Agency (FEMA) at www.fema.gov/pte/prep.htm

Emergency Sanitation: Federal Emergency Management Agency (FEMA) at www.fema.gov/library/sanitatf.htm

Food-Borne Illnesses: Impact of Lifestyles at
www.cdc.gov/ncidod/EID/vol3no4/collins.htm

Food and Drug Administration (FDA):
www.fda.gov

Food and Food Safety: Food and Drug
Administration/Center for Food Safety and Applied
Nutrition, Food, Nutrition, and Cosmetics Questions
and Answers at
www.vm.cfsan.fda.gov/~dms/qa-topin.html

Food Safety: Food and Drug Administration, The
Bad Bug Book at
www.vm.cfsan.fda.gov/~mow/intro.html

Food Safety List of Web Sites on WebCrawler.com at
www.webcrawler.com/health/for_professionals/med-
ical_specialties/public_health/food_safety

Food Safety Project, Iowa State University Extension:
www.extension.iastate.edu/foodsafety

Food Safety Sites Index, U.S. Department of
Agriculture:
www.nal.usda.gov/fnic/foodborne/fbindex/index.htm

Four Steps to Selecting a Child-Care Provider:
Administration for Children and Families, U.S.
Department of Health and Human Services at
www.acf.dhhs.gov/programs/ccb/faq/4steps.htm

Health, United States, 1999: National Center for
Health Statistics at
www.cdc.gov/nchs/products/pubs/pubd/hus/hus.htm

Resources

House Dust Mites:
www.allkids.org/Epstein/Articles/Dust_Mite.html and
www.ozemail.com.au/~lblanco

Immunization Schedule, U.S.: Centers for Disease
Control and Prevention at
www.cdc.gov/nip/recs/child-schedule.PDF

Institute for Food and Nutrition: www.ifst.org

Maternal and Child Health Bureau, Health
Resources and Services Administration, U.S.:
Department of Health and Human Services at
www.mchb.hrsa.gov

National Resource Center for Health and Safety in
Child Care: www.nrc.uchsc.edu

National Child Care Information Center (NCCIC):
www.nccic.org/statepro.html

National Food Safety Database:
www.foodsafety.org

Nosocomial Infections: Methicillin Resistant
Staphylococcus Aureus (MRSA) at
www.webcrawler.com/health/for_professionals/med
ical_specialties/public_health/environmental_health/
infection_control/?search=mrsa

Nosocomial Infections:
www.healthlinkusa.com/227.htm

Partnership for Food Safety Education Four Steps to
Fight Bac!: www.fightbac.org/steps/doubt.htm

Partnership for Food Safety Education:
www.fightbac.org/about/partners.htm

Ten Leading Causes of Death, Michigan and U.S.,
1998:
www.mdmh.state.mi.us/PHA/OSR/deaths/caus
rankcnty.asp

West Nile Encephalitis Virus: Centers for Disease
Control and Prevention at
www.cdc.gov/ncidod/dvbid/arbor/West_Nile_QA.htm

World Health Organization (WHO):
www.who.int

Zoonosis control: Diseases Transmitted from
Animals to Humans, Texas Department of Health at
www.r09.tdh.state.tx.us/zoonosis/zoonosis.html

Index

Index

305

Index

washing *(continued)*
  day care facilities and, 209–17,
    219
  nosocomial infections and,
    223–24, 226–30
  travel and, 231–32, 238–39,
    242
  see also soaps and detergents
water, 32, 94–107, 262, 265
  animals and, 188–89
  bioterrorism and, 248, 254
  bottled, 101–3, 243
  day care facilities and, 207–8
  distilled, 102–3

filtration of, 95–96, 98–103
harmful germs in, 96–97
location and purification of,
  105–7
repercussions of natural
disasters on, 104–7
from tap, 95–96, 99–101,
  236–37
travel and, 232, 235–43
from wells, 103–4, 106
West Nile virus, 10, 27,
  177, 185–87, 191

yeast, 35–36, 258–59, 261